12 Weeks to a Successful Data Dictionary

Maida Reavis Herbst, RRA

Opus Communications
Marblehead, MA

12 Weeks to a Successful Data Dictionary is published by Opus Communications.

Copyright 1997 by Opus Communications, Inc. All rights reserved. Printed in the United States of America.   5   4   3   2   1

ISBN 1-57839-000-1

Except where specifically encouraged, no part of this publication may be reproduced, in any form or by any means, without prior written consent of Opus Communications or the Copyright Clearance Center 508/750-8400. Please notify us immediately if you have received an unauthorized copy.

Opus Communications provides information resources for the health care industry. A select listing of our newsletters and books is found in the back of this book.

Jennifer I. Cofer, Publisher
Rob Stuart, Associate Publisher
Maida Reavis Herbst, Author
Jean St. Pierre, Art Director
Mike Kearney, Cover Design

Advice given is general. Readers should consult professional counsel for specific legal, ethical, or clinical questions. Arrangements can be made for quantity discounts.

For more information contact:

Opus Communications
P.O. Box 1168
Marblehead, MA 01945
Telephone: 800/650-6787 or 617/639-1872
Fax: 617/639-2982
E-mail: customer_service@opuscomm.com

Visit Opus Communications on the Web **http://www.opuscomm.com**

   All text pages are printed on recycled paper

Table of Contents

Preface ii

About the Author v

Introduction: The Information Age in Health Care 3

Chapter 1   What is A Data Dictionary, and Why Should You Build One? . 21

Chapter 2   Database Systems and Structures 33

Chapter 3   Setting Up the Team 43

Chapter 4   Meetings and Communications 59

Chapter 5   Planning and Designing the Data Dictionary 71

Chapter 6   Implementing the Data Dictionary 105

Chapter 7   Ongoing Development 125

Chapter 8   Case Study 137

Resources 145

A Glossary of Database Management Terms 147

Preface

Mention the words "data dictionary" in a health care setting and most people's eyes begin to glaze over. Speakers who attempt to discuss this topic at length are sure to lose their audience. What is it about data dictionaries that causes these reactions?

A data dictionary is a database of information about the data in various computer systems throughout the organization. Quite simply, it's a database about data. It contains basic data elements and gives detailed information about how each element is used in various databases. Most health care facilities have a multitude of computer systems with hundreds to thousands of data elements in each one. Just the idea of defining and cataloging all these data elements is overwhelming.

12 Weeks to a Successful Data Dictionary helps the non-technical reader apply a framework to the process of creating a data dictionary for a health care organization. Although portions of the process are highly technical, the person who is in charge of the data dictionary project does not need a strong technical background. A successful data dictionary requires wide participation throughout the organization, and relies not only on people who understand databases in great detail but also those who understand the importance of patient information and how it is used throughout the facility.

A data dictionary isn't built in a day; it's an evolutionary, step-by-step process that you should approach as if you were building an office structure. Select the site, draw up the plans, hire a contractor, prepare the site, build the foundation, frame the walls, and so on. The unique project plan in this book walks you through each step in the process.

12 Weeks to a Successful Data Dictionary divides the project into manageable segments. The introduction discusses the computer-based patient record (CPR)

and the importance of information management. Industry studies on the implementation of the CPR have set the price per hospital in a range from $2 million for a medium-sized facility to $40 million for a larger facility. Clearly, the establishment of a data dictionary is one of the least expensive tasks of CPR preparation. Chapter 1 addresses the rationale for data dictionaries and sets the stage for designing a project with a reasonable scope. Chapter 2 elaborates on database systems and structures for the nontechnical reader, and defines database management terms with a simple example.

This book uses a team approach to data dictionary development, as a collaborative process puts less of a burden on one person or department. Chapter 3 describes how to get support for the project and organize a team. Chapter 4 presents reminders on how to organize effective meetings and highlights techniques to improve communication among team members.

Chapters 5 and 6 describe a unique approach to the design and implementation of a data dictionary for a health care facility. You will design a data dictionary and begin to implement it. We outline a project of realistic size, develop a data dictionary model, and define a set of vital data elements. A starter set of data elements is provided using ASTM (American Society of Testing and Materials) standards and patient identification data elements.

Our data dictionary project can be accomplished within three months. By agreeing on a limited number of systems and a small set of data elements for the project, the organization is not overwhelmed; you can not only commit to the project but you can complete it. This completed project becomes a foundation upon which the organization continues to build. Chapter 7 outlines a plan to maintain and expand the data dictionary over the years. Chapter 8 is a case study of an organization that treats data as an important asset and weaves its data dictionary into the fabric of its data management plan.

Our approach to a data dictionary project applies to a variety of health care settings, including physician offices, hospitals, urgent care centers, long-term care facilities, mental health settings, and home health agencies. By building a data dictionary, not only do you comply with the JCAHO's IM.3 standard—uniformly define and capture data throughout your health care institution—but you also prepare your organization for the computerized patient record revolution.

Acknowledgments

The following people generously shared their expertise in databases, CPR, standards, and teamwork.

James R. Herbst
Deborah Kohn, MRH, RRA
Mary Fran Miller, MS, RRA
Gretchen Murphy, MEd, RRA
Sarah O'Gara, MPH, RRA
Roy Terry

Special thanks to the people from Holy Cross Health System Corporation for their cooperation in preparing the case study for this book.

Jean Balgrosky, RRA, MPH	Vice President, Information Resources
Hank Groot	Director of Decision Support Services
Gail Borlik	Database Administrator
Melanie Weller	Data Standards Analyst

M.R.H.

About the Author

Maida Reavis Herbst, RRA, has worked in health information management since 1981. She is co-owner of a health information management consulting company, Sunburst Information Management, Ltd., and is also employed by CodeMaster Cascade, a health information management software company. Ms. Herbst was previously Director of Medical Records at El Camino Hospital, the hospital with the distinction of having the first computerized clinical medical record system in the United States. She has served as president of the California Health Information Association (CHIA) and Technology Chair for both American Health Information Management Association and CHIA. Ms. Herbst has written numerous articles for state and national publications and has given presentations throughout the United States on data quality, data presentation, technology, health care reform, and computer-based patient records.

Introduction

The Information Age in Health Care

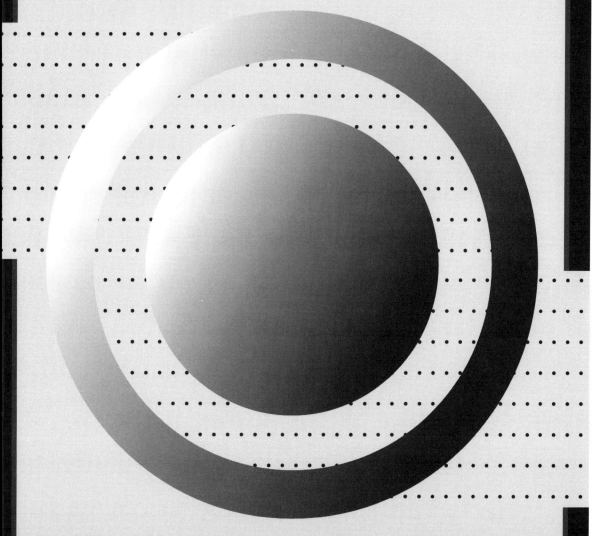

Introduction
The Information Age in Health Care

This decade is commonly called "The Information Age." Those who have and use information will enjoy a competitive advantage. The use of computers and networks has important implications, offering promise but also intense confusion; too many people confuse data with information.

Data is raw facts, figures, or observations. Information is data that has been processed and manipulated so that the results of the processing and manipulation are useful for decision-making and other organizational activities. To get meaningful information from its data resources, a business must have a strategic plan addressing its information needs and future business plans. The organization and use of information is vital for any business to thrive or survive.

This is especially true in the health care industry as it undergoes rapid change and tremendous growth. Patients spend less time in acute care settings and more time in ambulatory treatment centers; therefore inpatient length of stay is down and patient acuity is up. New medical technologies provide better diagnostic and treatment options. As the overall population grows and ages, there are more people needing more health care services.

Some of this change results from the move toward managed care, requiring health care providers to deliver quality care with fewer monetary resources. Not only must they practice efficiently, but they must prove that they have not diminished the quality of care. Health care facilities organize their internal data, analyze it, and report on selected outcomes to a variety of outside parties. With these demands for health care information on the increase, efficient methods are needed to move data and information from one computer system to another.

Facilities also need to share their data externally, as diverse health care services are being linked through multi-facility organizations and integrated delivery systems. Integrating the data of these diverse environments is expensive because each location typically has more than one computer system on a variety of hardware platforms, using a multitude of programming languages and software packages.

What types of computer systems exist in a typical health care organization? Most facilities have one main computer system running on a large mainframe. This serves as the core information system and processes the organization's main applications. Inpatient facilities have mainframes that are designed to capture and process financial information. Physician and clinic systems handle appointments and billings. Home health agencies, pharmacies, and reference laboratories use systems designed to handle their main business activities. Within each facility there are smaller departmental systems, some of which are capturing clinical data for patient care.

These stand-alone systems must now exchange data in order to provide meaningful information to clinicians for patient care and to administrators for outside reporting purposes. Linking financial data to clinical data allows a facility to track and review resource consumption, utilization, cost accounting, and case mix analysis. The ability to respond to purchaser (employer and health plans) demands makes an organization more attractive to consumers contracting for health care services.

The computer-based patient record

To no one's surprise, the landmark 1990 report from the Institute of Medicine (IOM) reported that paper-based medical records did not allow coordination of health care services within a facility or between other providers. The study determined that interfaces were poor between clinical data, administrative information, and medical knowledge and that health care providers could and should have better access to information to deliver better patient care. The study provided a blueprint for a computer-based patient record (CPR), also known as an electronic health record; it was envisioned that this CPR would be in a computer system that would support a variety of users by allowing them to access data, alerts, reminders, clinical decision support systems, and medical knowledge.

The IOM found no single system that could provide all these functions, but envisioned that the ultimate solution would not be a single entity like the older medical information systems, but rather an "open system" made up of building blocks of various applications that interface with each other or with a central clinical data repository or data warehouse.

The data dictionary

The study also noted that quality patient records MUST contain data that is meaningful for the users. The retrieval and use of information is presently limited by inconsistencies in the way that findings, problems, medications, and other data are named. The study recommended the use of a common clinical data dictionary and clinical codification systems that would produce uniform data for complete and reliable analysis of patient care and disease trends. A data dictionary is essentially an ordered collection of data that describes and locates each data element in an information system. The data dictionary is a key component of the CPR, as will be demonstrated in subsequent chapters.

A common and effective way to manage the exchange of data between computer systems is the use of an "interface engine." This is commercial or "home grown" software and the associated hardware that coordinates the exchange of data between different computer platforms. All departmental systems send data to the interface engine and it, in turn, passes data back to other systems. The interface engine acts like a translator, converting data to the format needed by the computer system that receives the data. Obviously, managing interfaces demands a data dictionary that explicitly defines how data must be transformed before exchanging.

Data capture

Now, just a few years after the IOM released their report, the CPR is beginning to unfold as they envisioned it. More and more data is captured in electronic form and stored in a variety of systems. The data sources include physicians, nurses, therapists, technicians, computer monitoring devices, and even the patients themselves.

Each type of data is captured in a variety of ways. It can be generated from computer monitoring devices, keyboarded into a computer, or entered via touch-screen, light pen, or mouse. Information is stored in a variety of ways, including paper output, film images, tracings, computer disk, optical storage, video, and sound. All this data is analyzed differently within the computer systems, interpreted in a variety of ways by clinicians, technicians, and administrators, and then transformed into information. This information is used in clinical decision-making, patient education, research, organizational decision-making, and performance improvement. Together, these integrated data form the information resources of a health care facility.

Data integration
Integration allows improved access to clinical information by clinicians throughout the health care system and it also allows for improved analysis of clinical and financial data. Clinical data repositories capture data from many other application systems and are the central database for clinical information. Even bigger databases, called data warehouses, store masses of clinical and financial information; this provides one central location for all transaction data where users can make requests and receive summarized information. Like the CPR, these central data repositories and data warehouses may not reside on one system or in one location. Data may be stored on different hardware systems, using separate operating systems and different languages, but the key is that users can access the data as if it were located on a single system; the complexity of a data warehouse is hidden from the users.

This causes many issues and problems for information designers and information users. There are multiple input sources. There is the potential to overwrite information with a subsequent data entry. Some users should be allowed to update, some to delete, and some to do both; electronic rights for various functions need to be specified. Changes in regulations may force changes to system rules and structure. The same data element, for instance PATIENT NAME, exists in many systems. Redundant data costs money and, if not managed properly, this redundancy will be magnified with the addition of each new computer system. An effective data dictionary in a well-designed database system eliminates redundancy through the use of data relationships. DATE OF BIRTH, for instance, no longer needs to be stored in multiple locations when a data dictionary catalogs the location of DATE OF BIRTH in the ADT (admission/discharge/transfer) system and links all of the patient information through the medical record number.

Standards for information management

We are now struggling to automate a trillion dollar industry and we do not have universal information management standards. Health care information professionals must take part in the planning and development of new computer systems that can support the CPR and the unification of health care information. Not only must they do this within their institutions but they must also reference emerging standards that can assist in guiding the content and structure of electronic health care records. This will assist in promoting consistency between systems and organizations and it will allow reliable, efficient data transfer.

In the health care environment, the term "standard" includes guidelines developed by federal and state governments, accrediting agencies, and professional agencies and trade associations. These standards encourage or require conformance with set values, measurements, or guidelines. The development of standards for the CPR has been ponderous because of the overwhelming size of the project. The electronic advances in the banking and insurance industries, for example, have outstripped the progress made in the health care industry because their applications and products are so much simpler.

Health care facilities are like miniature towns, engaging in a wide variety of commercial activities. Besides the main activity, patient care, health care facilities also do a lot of banking, provide laundry and transportation services, and serve food to patients and employees. Developing standards for this wide variety of services is overwhelming. Standards development for the health care industry has been largely "catch as catch can," with government assistance only when it concerns the government (eg, Medicare billing) or when trade organizations will benefit (regional data projects).

Before the exchange of clinical data can occur, systems must agree on what is being transferred back and forth. Many vendors and some government agencies have developed their own internal data dictionaries. These dictionary definitions vary from system to system; they have different data elements with varying names and relationships between them. One vendor calls a field GENDER and another vendor refers to it as SEX. Valid entries for this field are "male" and "female" in the lab system, "M" and "F" in the pharmacy system, and "1" and "2" in the billing system. These inconsistent naming conventions and encoding schemes cause nightmares for information systems people who try to move data between systems. This is where standardization comes in.

Standards development agencies

There are various standards development agencies working to develop recommended standards, policies, and practices in four major areas: clinical and medical data sets, eligibility determination, provider location, and patient confidentiality and privacy. The major standards groups include HL7, ANSI, ASTM, ASC X12, WEDI, and IEEE (see Table A on page 11). These groups promote the development of voluntary standards, developed through a consensus process. Various vendors, health care professionals, and other private and public sector organizations are participating in this work.

Health care institutions will benefit by referring to these national standards and promoting their use in the data dictionary. By using these standards, a facility enables the exchange of information that can be compared in meaningful ways between health care systems, or in a Community Health Information Network (CHIN) or Regional Health Information Network (RHIN).

Most CHINs and RHINs propose to use online information technologies to allow health care organizations, providers, purchasers, consumers, researchers, and policy-makers to exchange clinical and administrative data electronically, and in a paperless environment. CHINs and RHINs require the use of information systems that abide by common standards. They encourage the streamlining and sharing of information and the reduction of redundancy of data by contending that the community health status will be improved. Their goal is to track patient care information over a lifetime. This is the information-age equivalent of having a family physician who delivers patients, treats them during childhood and adulthood, and attends to them during old age.

JCAHO's IM *standards*

In 1994, the Joint Commission on Accreditation of Healthcare Organizations (JCAHO) developed ten new standards under the heading of Management of Information. These standards mainly address inpatient facilities, but they provide a template for understanding information management across all health care settings. The information management standards challenge health care organizations to take a facility-wide approach to information management by stipulating timely and easy access to information throughout the health care facility. When an organization manages its information assets well, it has more accurate information that can be used for quality improvement activities—a key process in any business. When information is well organized it can also be shared by all users throughout the facility.

The JCAHO Information Management (IM) standards address four major types of information to be managed in a health care facility: patient-specific (ie, patients' medical records), aggregate information (usually stored in databases), expert knowledge–based (found under medical library services), and comparative (for quality improvement, research, and administrative uses). This book addresses the first category, patient-specific types of information.

The IM standards outline that an IM planning process is designed to meet the health care organization's internal and external information needs. Each organization assesses its needs for information management based on its mission, goals, services, personnel, mode(s) of service delivery (ie, hospital, home care, ambulatory), resources, and access to affordable technology. Addressing confidentiality, security, integrity, and timeliness of access are also important IM tasks.

The third standard, IM.3, states "Uniform data definitions and methods for capturing data are in place when feasible." IM.3 challenges a facility to uniformly define and capture data throughout the entire health care facility. This standard can be fulfilled by establishing a data dictionary that, in brief, catalogs who is responsible for collecting data, how the data is collected, who uses it, and who can change it. The data dictionary should be maintained in a database, as discussed in Chapter 2. Through this process, in addition to having an organized system that provides information about the facility's data, redundancies, inconsistencies, and omissions are identified.

Minimum data sets

Over the years, data has been submitted to various governmental, public, and private bodies. These are commonly known as "minimum data sets." Their use promotes uniform data collection and reporting. The most common data set is called the Uniform Hospital Discharge Data Set (UHDDS). This was developed by the U.S. Department of Health, Education and Welfare in 1974 to establish a core set of data elements to be used in reporting for Medicare and Medicaid programs (see Table B on page 15). There are minimum data sets for other clinical settings such as ambulatory medicine, home care, hospice, long-term care, occupational health, and emergency medicine. Other common data sets like the UB-92 and HCFA 1500 standardize the claims process. There is a similarity between this type of data submission and the development and use of a data dictionary because each data element is defined so that aggregate information is meaningful. Guidelines for these data sets are periodically updated by the responsible party, eg, HCFA.

Minimum data sets were early attempts at data standardization. Now that health care is moving into the information age, we have computer-assisted aids to help us get ready for computerized patient records. This book can help you move from data disorganization to information management through the use of a powerful tool, a data dictionary.

TABLE A - Standards Organizations	
ANSI (American National Standards Institute)	Formed in 1918 as the coordinating body for voluntary standards for fields such as information technology to building construction within the US.
ASC X12 (Accredited Standards Committee)	Formed by ANSI in 1979 as a subcommittee, this is the organization for developing, publishing, and maintaining standards of electronic data interchange for insurance enrollment, eligibility, and claims payment.
ASTM (American Society for Testing and Materials)	Created in 1898 as a forum for producers and consumers to develop uniform standards for products, materials, systems, and services.
ASTM Committee E-31 on Computerized Systems	Selected subcommittees include Computer-based Patient Records, Clinical Laboratory Systems, Clinical Observations, Health Data Cards, Medical Transcription, Pharmacy, and Health Information Networks.
CEN	Comite European de Normalisation. "The ECC has a community-wide organization to develop standards. TC 251 is developing an integrated set of standards for use in healthcare. CEN is interested in cooperating and coordinating with US efforts but will develop a divergent approach with concrete forms for cooperation and sharing experience."

TABLE A - Standards Organizations (continued)	
CPRI	Founded at the recommendation of the Institute of Medicine Committee on Improving the Patient Record. The mission is to initiate and coordinate activities facilitating and promoting the use of computer-based patient records. Membership includes health care payers, providers, information technology companies, and health care associations.
DICOM (Digital Imaging and Communications in Medicine)	Develops standards used in the exchange of diagnostic images including MRI scans, x-rays, CT scans, nuclear medicine, and ultrasound images and for electronic exchange between diagnostic equipment from different manufacturers.
HISB (Healthcare Informatics Standards Board)	Formed in 1991 as an ANSI subcommittee and composed of both individual and corporate members, it is the official coordinating body for all US health care standards developers responsible for setting informatics standards and coordinating standards for the US.
HL7 (Health Level Seven)	Formed in 1987 to develop standards for the interchange of clinical, financial, and administrative data through hospital information systems, clinical laboratory systems, enterprise systems, and pharmacy systems. Their application protocol for electronic data interchange is the standard used by a majority of health care system vendors.

TABLE A - Standards Organizations (continued)	
HL7 (Health Level Seven) (continued)	Application protocol for electronic data exchange of key sets of data swapped between different application systems in health care environments. Facilitate data sharing among application systems. Cross-vendor clinical information sharing.
IEEE (Institute of Electrical and Electronics Engineers)	"A family of standards that provides for inter connectivity and interoperability of medical devices and hospital information systems."
ISO (International Organization for Standardization)	A non-governmental worldwide federation of national standards bodies formed in 1947 and based in Geneva, Switzerland, with 2,700 technical committees, subcommittees, and working groups charged with resolving global standardization problems. Some subcommittees are devoted exclusively to healthcare, such as transfusion and injection devices, dentistry, anesthetic and respiratory equipment, prosthetics and orthotics, sterilization, and clinical lab testing systems.
NII (National Information Infrastructure)	A Denver private sector organization founded in 1993 and charged with CPR and telemedicine data infrastructure information exchange via the nationwide electronic data network.

TABLE A - Standards Organizations (continued)	
WEDI (Workgroup for Electronic Data Interchange)	Organization whose mission is to promote health care electronic commerce and connectivity and that is made up of providers, payers, government agencies, standards-setting organizations, vendors, and consumer organizations.

TABLE B - UHDDS Data Set	
DATA ELEMENT	**DEFINITION**
1. Personal Identification	The unique number assigned to each patient within the hospital that distinguishes the patient and his or her hospital record from all others in that institution
2. Date of Birth	Month, day, and year of birth
3. Sex	Male or female
4a. Race	White, Black, Asian or Pacific Islander, American Indian/Eskimo/Aleut, other
4b. Ethnicity	Spanish origin/Hispanic, Non-Spanish origin/Non-Hispanic
5. Residence	Zip code, code for foreign residence
6. Hospital Identification	A unique institutional number within a data collection system
7 - 8. Admission and Discharge Dates	Month, day, and year of both admission and discharge
9 - 10. Physician Identification	Each physician must have a unique identification number within the hospital. The attending physician and the operating physician (if applicable) are to be identified.

TABLE B - UHDDS Data Set (continued)	
Attending Physician	The clinician who is primarily and largely responsible for the care of the patient from the beginning of the hospital episode.
Operating Physician	The clinician who performed the principal procedure.
11. Diagnoses	All diagnoses that affect the current hospital stay.
a. Principal Diagnosis	The condition established after study to be chiefly responsible for occasioning the admission of the patient to the hospital for care.
b. Other Diagnoses	All conditions that coexist at the time of admission, that develop subsequently, or that affect the treatment received and/or the length of stay. Diagnoses that related to an earlier episode which have no bearing on the current hospital stay are to be excluded.
12. Procedures and Date	All significant procedures are to be reported.
a. Significant Procedure	A procedure that is: 1. Surgical in nature 2. Carries a procedural risk 3. Carries an anesthetic risk 4. Requires specialized training

	TABLE B - UHDDS Data Set (continued)
b. Identity and Date	For significant procedures, the identity (by unique number within the hospital) of the person performing the procedure and the date must be reported.
c. Principal procedure	One that was performed for definitive treatment rather than one performed for diagnostic or exploratory purposes, or was necessary to take care of a complication. If there appear to be two procedures that are principal, then the one most related to the principal diagnosis would be selected as the principal procedure.
13. Disposition of Patient	Discharged to home (routine) Left against medical advice Discharged to another short-term hospital Discharged to a long-term care institution Died Other
14. Expected Payer for Most of This Bill	Single major source that the patient expects will pay for his or her bill Blue Cross Other insurance companies Medicare Medicaid Workers' Compensation Other government payers

TABLE B - UHDDS Data Set (continued)	
14. Expected Payer for Most of This Bill (continued)	Self-pay No charge (free, charity, special research, or teaching) Other

Chapter 1
What is A Data Dictionary, and Why Should You Build One?

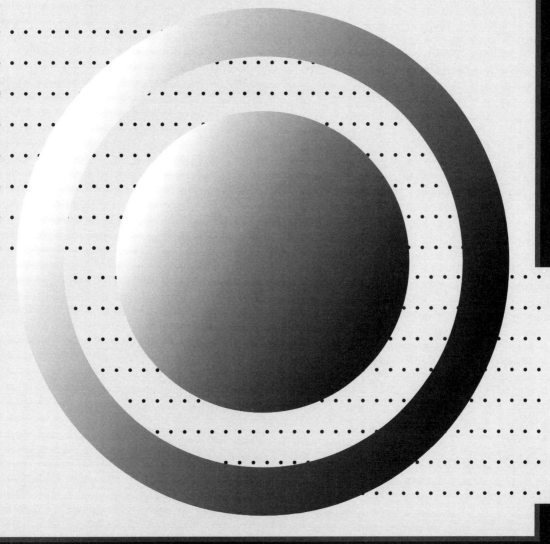

Chapter 1
What is a Data Dictionary, and Why Should You Build One?

There are a variety of methodologies for assembling a data dictionary but no how-to guides giving practical advice for building one in a health care organization. This book is such a guide, and provides an outline for a data dictionary project with a defined scope.

Attacking the data dictionary as a project has the benefit of providing well-defined starting and ending dates, clear objectives, and a set schedule and budget. The project will be completed within a 12-week period and will not exceed a budget of $18,500. After the project ends, the data dictionary grows as the information systems department and departments with clinical computer systems continue to add data elements to it. This 12-week method is used because building a data dictionary in a health care facility can be an overwhelming prospect. Many facilities start out with the best of intentions but soon become mired in the difficulty of agreeing on standard terminology, or they become overwhelmed with the sheer volume of data elements.

A motivating reason for an institution to build a data dictionary is to effectively organize its information resources; this is a prerequisite to the implementation of a truly integrated computerized patient record (CPR). Information is made up of individual pieces of data that have been manipulated so that the results are useful for decision-making and other organizational activities. This manipulated data is more available to users when it is accessible through a database and associated software.

Databases
Database systems and structures are discussed more fully in Chapter 2 but, briefly, a database is defined as a storage location for all user data. Moreover, it is an interrelated collection of data that is shared by organization users and is

designed to meet the needs of the users and the organization. A well-structured database reduces data redundancy and increases uniformity and accessibility to information. There are fewer errors and variability in reports generated from an organized database.

Data dictionaries

A data dictionary is a database of information about the data in various computer systems throughout the organization. Quite simply, it's a database about data. It contains basic data elements and gives detailed information about how each element is used in various databases. For example, the term "patient name" seems simple enough to the users who input it into a computer, yet in building a data dictionary, the team is likely to find that one department lists last name first while another department lists first name first; one department may list the middle initial while another gives the full middle name. What's more, one database may allow 33 characters for name, while another allows 28 characters.

Some of the common elements a data dictionary could define include

- Patient Name,
- Previously Registered Name,
- Patient Number,
- Social Security Number,
- Date and Time of Birth,
- Sex,
- Occupation,
- Patient Address, and
- Home Phone.

Some of the detailed information, or attributes, that should appear in the definition of each element include format type (eg, number or date), number of characters, synonyms, and password protection level. For a detailed description of these attributes for patient name, see Table 5E in Chapter 5.

Simple or complex

A very simple data dictionary can be created using a word processor. Using this approach, a facility would alphabetically catalog all of the various computer system's data elements and their attributes. This list would be improved by putting it in table format so that new data elements could be inserted in proper order. Some facilities have such a data dictionary, but the major drawbacks are that very few people can access it, no reports can be generated from it, and it is often not current. A library index card system would work better than this.

On the other hand, a data dictionary that is maintained in a computerized database allows a health care facility to visually represent the relationships between its computer systems and give its users a structured format for exchanging information about data organization. It also allows users to query the data dictionary in a variety of ways. If a health care system is merging previously independent facilities, a user might be designing a corporate MPI and would query the data dictionary database (DDDB) asking to see all systems that have a field called MEDICAL RECORD NUMBER. Another user could be linking a new system in a clinical data repository and would query the DDDB asking for a list of all data elements in the new system. This sort of system is easy to use, provides information to requesters, and is therefore well maintained. In Chapters 5 and 6 you will learn how to build just such a database over a 12-week period.

Passive or active

Data dictionaries can be either passive or active. The passive type is designed as a reference tool for the users of data and is not directly linked to any application system. A passive data dictionary database resides in a software program but does not interface or connect with the computer systems it is defining. The active type always resides in a software program and directs the various database systems to obtain data items. It directs the data traffic and knows where data are stored, who has access to them, what their values are, and various other characteristics. Either type of data dictionary can be set up to perform edits and validate data entry. For example, if a registrar attempts to enter a patient's last name with a hyphen and hyphens are not valid, the data dictionary will not allow the registrar to proceed until the format is correct.

When a user queries a passive data dictionary for a list of all systems that have the data item MEDICAL RECORD NUMBER, the response is a listing of all the systems that contain this field or any other field defined as MEDICAL RECORD NUMBER (synonyms include PATIENT NUMBER, CHART NUMBER, etc.). A request to an active data dictionary is more specific because the user obtains a specific patient's medical record number from all the various systems that contain that patient's medical record number and all of the data associated with those records.

Why build one?

In an ideal world, data elements in one computer system would exactly match the same data elements in another computer system. DATE OF BIRTH would be standardized with a format of, for instance, MMDDYYYY. Health care organizations, though, are made up of many systems designed by competing vendors with little incentive to standardize. Designing and implementing a data dictionary gives a health care organization the opportunity to build a tool that allows for close investigation of how the different computer systems function. You can design a data dictionary to accept multiple definitions and formats for each data element and to include pointers to standard definitions. You cannot realistically force standardization on an entire facility, but you can document how each computer system is set up and build pointers to standardized definitions.

This kind of data dictionary helps an organization maintain consistent databases across the enterprise. As an organization acquires and creates new computer systems, there are clear guidelines to follow as the data components are developed. The data dictionary allows standardization for multi-vendor workstations and lets users display, analyze, and report on consistent, accurate data. This scenario fits the definition of a CPR—an open system of various applications that provides useful information to many types of users.

Integrity and uniformity

To be truly useful, health care information must be accurate. Health care providers will avoid using any information they do not think is reliable, valid, or complete. For example, a medical clinic uses Current Procedural Terminology (CPT) to code immunizations. The coding is usually done in the billing department by people who quickly review super bills sent down from the physicians' offices. If a Quality Improvement department pulls immunization statistics from this billing information (which is often ill-defined, inaccurate, and incomplete), the clinicians will quickly point out that the numbers are wrong. They will use these poor statistics to combat every effort made to try to prove that their immunization rates are too low.

Data must be collected uniformly using standardized and structured codification systems. If there is more than one single set of data definitions, the data is unusable for any type of aggregate study. There are multiple opportunities to misinterpret medical data, including poor quality source documents, variable practitioner terminology, and plain old human error. Why complicate matters with multiple, inconsistent data definitions?

Accessibility and timeliness

Accessibility to clinical data is currently monitored by documenting dictated report turnaround time, chart availability, or chart completion statistics. A different spin on accessibility and timeliness is to ask "how do the information systems serve the clinicians?"—in other words, can they enter data and access information in a way that is immediate and helpful for better patient care? When a clinician wants a list of all patients under five years old treated for a fever of unknown origin over the past five years, is that information immediately available? Could the clinician request that information from a computer terminal without assistance? Would it include those patients seen in both the clinic and the urgent care center?

Providers make entries in the medical record and receive information from each other's entries. A CPR must be designed for use by the clinicians but it must ultimately be easier to use than paper. Immediate accessibility to other care providers' entries and to test results would give any clinician an incentive to learn the computer system. Standard data definitions form the foundation of a system that is accessible and simple to understand.

Integration

Increased computerization in health care facilities means that there is an increased need for communication between systems. Multiple systems are being interfaced and integrated to improve the speed and flow of clinical data. Whether your plan is to eventually replace existing systems with a "super" system, to link systems, or to store key data in a central repository, developing a data dictionary will benefit you in all cases. It is the building block for all of these approaches to improving communications between systems. When data definitions are in place, systems can communicate and share information. A data dictionary is a tool that can be used to control discrepancies in the meaning and naming of data elements.

Systems integration also means a reduction of redundant data collection efforts. Documentation of data elements through the use of a data dictionary encourages the sharing of data resources, because the users of the data understand where data originates, what the validations and edits are, and who has control of the data. This ultimately contributes to a reduction in the cost of computerization. Not only are data elements gathered fewer times, but they are also efficiently stored. How many times are allergies documented? If they are documented in one place, accessible through interfaces across all systems, it's all the same to the end user—they can still get to the information they need.

Patient identification data elements are another good example. Every computer system has a location for the demographic data elements that uniquely identify patients. There are even separate Master Patient Index (MPI) systems, which are stand-alone or part of the Registration/ADT (Admission/Discharge/Transfer) system. The MPI is designed to ensure that identification and demographic information is accurate and consistent across systems, that information uniquely identifying a patient is available for subsequent encounters, and that all the information about the patient is available for clinical, administrative, and reimbursement purposes. Standardizing the MPI data elements ensures that interfaced computers can share this important information.

Clinical data management
The mission of any health care facility is to provide effective, efficient, quality patient care services. Good information management will assist the facility in meeting this mission. Information management should be planned around a health care facility's needs based on the setting (eg, ambulatory, long-term care, inpatient) or the types of services it offers (eg, home health, IV therapy, physical therapy, trauma). The end result, in all cases, should be to coordinate clinical data and make it available to users throughout the organization.

Additionally, clinical data must be well organized so it is available for reporting and comparison purposes. Clinicians need diagnostic information about current and past treatment of patients; they need to obtain information about how similar patient groups responded to different therapies. Managed care dictates that physician and hospital peer comparisons are made using information obtained from within the facility and comparing it with information from outside. Physicians in one region are being compared with their peers in another region using c-section and VBAC (vaginal birth after c-section) rates. Process improvement takes place through analysis of case management, the use of critical paths, and practice guidelines. Treatment modalities and interventions need to be analyzed. Orthopedic physicians are interested in analyzing the variances in patients who have had total joint replacements. In order to fulfill these requests and to generate reports, the data elements must be structured. This structure can be provided through the use of a data dictionary.

Scope of project
Succinctly stated, the objective of the project in this book is to implement a passive database data dictionary for a core set of data elements and eight designated departments using ASTM standards. The implementation helps

demonstrate compliance with the JCAHO IM.3 Standard and to begin to standardize data in preparation for the implementation of a CPR.

Whether you are building a data dictionary to comply with the JCAHO IM.3 Standard or you are readying your facility for the CPR, you are embarking on an interesting adventure. When you build a data dictionary, you develop a vocabulary of meaningful concepts that will assist people in solving problems about electronic communication. As you extend the project across the institution, you assist people in understanding how others define their view of the organization.

This undertaking requires at least a working knowledge of databases; this topic is reviewed briefly in Chapter 2. Building a data dictionary in a facility of any size is a group project; special skills are required to ensure that a group of people move together in the same direction, and in the same time frame. Setting up your team and organizing communications and meetings are discussed in Chapters 3 and 4. Planning, designing, and implementing the data dictionary are covered in Chapters 5 and 6. Suggestions about how to keep your data dictionary alive and growing are found in Chapter 7. Chapter 8 presents a case study of a health care system that is in the process of adding to its corporate data dictionary.

Before you begin this project you must understand that a data dictionary is never "done." If you "finish," it is a good sign that you and your organization are no longer using your data dictionary. For example, acute care hospitals have been required for years to have an approved abbreviation list. This list is usually developed under the auspices of the Medical Record Committee through the work of the Health Information Department. Many of the abbreviations are taken from medical reference books and do not accurately reflect the abbreviations actually used in the facility. The approved list may be pulled out, dusted off, and somewhat updated just before the next accreditation inspection, but the rest of the time it languishes in a binder and people rarely refer to it.

A data dictionary is a powerful tool, and with an online data dictionary there will be continued additions, changes, and deletions as systems grow and transform. The goal of this book is to get you started on building a data dictionary that will be referred to and used by the various requesters of health care information. You will organize one of your institution's most precious resources—information.

Notes

Chapter 2
Database Systems and Structures

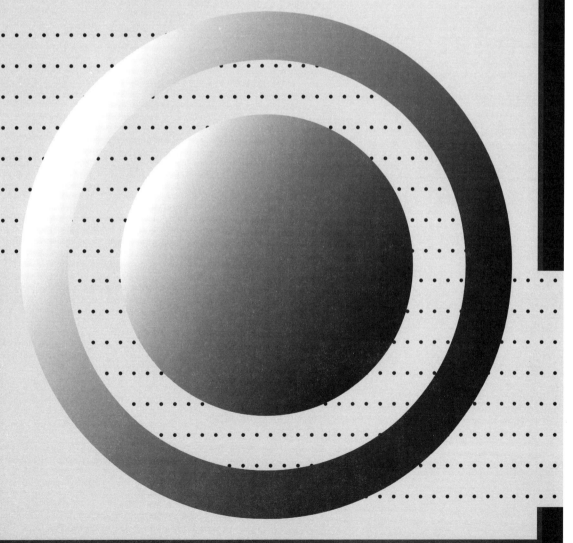

Chapter 2
Database Systems and Structures

If you have at least a basic understanding of databases, you can skip to Chapter 3 to learn how to set up your project team. If you do not know much about databases, this chapter will give you a broad overview and an appreciation for how a database is used in a data dictionary project. You'll also learn the importance of designing a data dictionary that meets the needs of your Information Systems (IS) department and the computer users throughout your organization.

Database types

The databases in a health care institution may be flat-file, network, hierarchical, relational, or object-oriented. A typical health care facility probably has two or more of these designs existing in different departments. We will briefly discuss two traditional types, flat file and hierarchical systems. We will then define and illustrate relational databases with an example at the end of this chapter.

Traditional systems

Until the advent of the relational model, data processing applications routinely used flat file systems. "Flat file" is the industry term for a plain text file where data is organized in rows and columns. Traditional application programs are designed to read data from files that are organized in a given row and column format. Often the data files belong to a single department or function of the organization and are not available to others. The data is very closely integrated with the program that uses it.

An example of a flat file is a health information system that stores all the UHDDS data elements for each patient in separate rows. The data elements for each patient are stored in a specific location, depending on the data element. One patient has 5 diagnoses and 3 procedures; another patient has 15 diagnoses and no procedures. The flat file structure has 15 diagnosis slots and 10 procedure slots allocated to each record; in this example there are 10 empty diagnosis slots and 7 empty procedure slots in the first record and all the diagnosis slots are full and procedure slots empty in the second example. This type of file organization requires a huge amount of data redundancy.

Hierarchical systems were the next advance in database processing. In this type of system, information is still organized in files, but the relationship between files is defined as "parent-child." For example, the Order File is related to the Laboratory File as its child. An application program is written so that once a patient record is selected from the Laboratory File all associated order records for that patient will be selected and available. The problem with this file structure is that it is difficult or even impossible to report only orders without accessing the patient records.

Relational systems

A relational database is one that is designed to store and retrieve shared and related data. This is considered the current state of the art in database design. The evolving type of database, called "object oriented," is not covered in this book. In a relational system there are at least two and possibly hundreds of tables of data consisting of rows and columns. Each table is a collection of data about a particular subject such as patient medications, physician lists, or inventory supply itemizations. Tables are linked to each other through one common data element so that data can be combined in just about any way the user needs it, yet redundancy (storing the same data element in more than one place) is minimized. An example of a relational file structure appears at the end of this chapter.

User group

Without users, there would be no need for the database. In a health care organization, this user group is made up of all the departments that generate, process, or use data. Some departments may be fairly low-end users, such as laundry, requiring only minimal information and having noncritical needs. Other departments may constantly use the systems and have critical needs, such as pharmacy, radiology, and the patient accounts office. They heavily rely on the organization's computing resources. Chapter 3 addresses how to approach the users in a health care organization.

IS infrastructure

IS has authority for defining and enforcing data standards. They have to approve all changes to data standards. Moreover, IS must provide support to nontechnical users if the data dictionary implementation is to be successful.

Overall responsibility for the database rests with a database administrator. This person is responsible for organizing the information resources, tuning the database, and efficiently splitting the tables to give quick access and error recovery.

Unless you are very comfortable with the design and use of databases, you should call on the expertise of a database administrator to provide expert advice on choosing the right type of database. In addition, an administrator can assist you with the technical portions of analyzing, designing, and implementing a data dictionary in a database. This will save you time and dramatically lower the learning curve for you and the other team members.

Queries

How do users access all this organized data? They use queries. Queries are requests made to the database, such as "Show me all patients whose payment source is Medicare." The data that answers the query can be from one table, or from many tables, but the query brings the information together in one location for the user. The set of records that a query brings back is known as a dynaset or a subset.

The users are completely shielded from the underlying complexity, as the answer to a query may pull together fields from three or four different tables into the user view. Pharmacy needs to view the patient address combined with prescribed medication doses and prescribing physician. A pharmacist's "view" would show all this information on one screen. Unbeknownst to the pharmacist, however, the patient address would be in a different table in the database than the dosage information and the physician name.

On the other hand, a case manager's view may show the same address information but would include the patient's phone number for a follow-up telephone call instead of the medication information seen by the pharmacist.

DBMS

Each database contains software that manages and controls the data. This database management system (DBMS), along with a human database administrator, manages the data by

- creating computerized database files,
- managing additions of data to the file,
- altering data in the file,
- organizing the data,
- providing query languages,
- allowing multi-user access,
- retrieving data in response to queries,
- enforcing security (user log-ons, passwords, record access restrictions), and
- maintaining an audit trail or log of all activities.

User requests are interpreted and processed by the DBMS. Physical management, tracking, and verification is also done by the DBMS. Lastly, the software relationship between data fields is managed by the DBMS. A DBMS allows a user to enter, change, organize, locate, retrieve, and sort data. The end result of this work is the creation of useful information.

Database example

It can be difficult to communicate with colleagues immersed in the field of database management. With all this discussion of database systems and structures, a pictorial example should bring the point home. Let's take a look at a relational database model. Some of the key concepts to understand are described below and in the glossary at the end of the book. This is as technical as this book gets, so look at the example and hang on until the end of the chapter.

Rows and columns

The data in a database table is arranged in columns (called fields) and rows (called records). One data record contains all the specified facts about one "data entity" in that table. For instance, in a table of patient-identifying information, a row would contain all data for only one patient such as patient number, patient name, sex, date of birth, etc. The columns (or "fields") represent the types of data gathered for each row (or "record").

The field is a category of information also known as an attribute and the row is known as a tuple; the intersection of a row and a column contains a data value. In the Master Patient Index Table (see Table 2A), the first field is the PATIENT NO. (or medical record number), the next field is PATIENT NAME, then SEX, DATE OF BIRTH, and SSAN (social security number).

A record is a collection of information about one person, place, thing, or event. In this table, the first row contains identifying information about Monica A. Harold. This row is defined as a "record" and is the area in the database that organizes identifying information about Monica A. Harold.

Keys

Each record in the table contains the same set of fields and each field has the same type of information for each record. If you have more than one table, they

TABLE 2A - Master Patient Index Table

Patient No.	Patient Name	Sex	Date of Birth	SSAN
5490300	Harold, Monica A	F	12/03/25	000-00-0000
3982688	Rodriquez, Henry G	M	08/30/55	000-00-0001
0984585	Nguyen, Tran B	M	11/24/67	000-00-0002
0874587	Gee, Amy R	F	05/16/77	000-00-0003
1939574	Martins, Robert I	M	09/09/21	000-00-0004

are cross referenced (related) to each other through the use of keys. A "key" is a data item that is used to identify a record in a database table. A "primary key" is a data item that uniquely identifies a record; a "secondary key" does not uniquely identify but identifies a number of records in a set that share the same properties. In the Master Patient Index Table, the primary key is PATIENT NO.

In the Financial Table example (see Table 2B), the primary key is also PATIENT NO. These primary keys establish the relationship between tables and provide indices to data contained in records (rows). This allows the software to search the database efficiently and quickly. Tables can also contain secondary keys, eg, in the Master Patient Index Table, PATIENT NAME is a secondary key. These keys allow related records in different tables to be linked together.

A departmental database may contain hundreds of tables with many columns of information. A large organizational database probably contains thousands of tables. When the user requests information from the database, the software accesses various tables using the relationships between them. In the case of a request for a list of names, ages, and sex of all patients with Medicare insurance, the database search would first run through the Financial Table, finding all records with a PAYMENT SOURCE of Medicare and then would use the primary key, PATIENT NO., as an index to the desired information in the Master

TABLE 2B - Financial Table

Patient No.	Payment Source	Payor ID No
5490300	Medicare	000000033
3982688	Blue Cross	000000031
0984585	Blue Shield	000000030
0874587	Medicaid	000000032
1939574	Medicare	000000033

Patient Index Table. The query would then retrieve PATIENT NAME and SEX and would also compute age from the current date and the DATE OF BIRTH. It would then add this to the request and display a user view, in this case a list such as that seen in Table 2C.

TABLE 2C - Results of a Request for a List of Patients with Medicare				
Patient No.	**Patient Name**	**Patient Age**	**Sex**	**Payment Source**
5490300	Harold, Monica A	70	F	Medicare
1939574	Martins, Robert I	76	M	Medicare

Congratulations! You made it through the complicated database example and have finished the most technical chapter of the book. It is important that you understand how databases work because a data dictionary functions best if it is built in a database. With this level of detail accomplished, we can get back to the project at hand and create a data dictionary. The next step is to organize the team necessary to embark on the project.

Notes

Chapter 3
Setting Up the Team

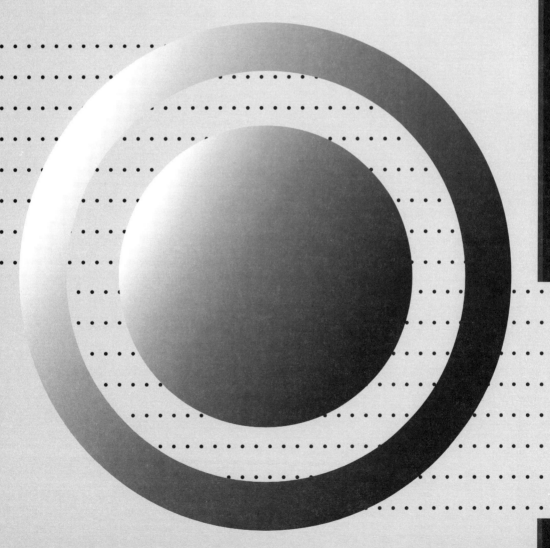

Chapter 3
Setting Up the Team

Creating the right team is a key step in the data dictionary project. In a project of this scope and size, one person cannot accomplish the task alone. Whether you choose to have three or thirty team members, the success of the project will depend on what the members of the team produce, both independently and cooperatively. Remember, the goal is to organize your health care facility's information resources by developing a data dictionary.

Project support

Getting a data dictionary project off to a good start requires good preparation and homework. The first steps include ensuring that the organization can make this a priority, garnering strong support for the project, and getting the time, labor, and money it will require.

Making the project a priority

To make the project a priority, you must clarify the purpose for the data dictionary, its end use and benefits. People on all levels will participate more willingly and actively if they can understand why something is needed and what the consequences of not having it are. The Introduction and Chapter 1 provided a strong rationale for developing a data dictionary. This included

- development of the CPR,
- integration of data,
- consolidation of information resources,
- management of clinical information, and
- availability of data for patient care.

Use these convincing arguments to present a clear picture of your project and the benefits to the facility.

You must be aware of other activities that may get the data dictionary project off track. There are external factors that can impact the project. You may work in an inpatient facility that is merging with a large clinic nearby, or you may work for a home health agency that is being acquired by a national company. If this is the case, you should rethink your time frame for implementation so it does not conflict with system-wide initiatives; your facility's top priority will be the reorganization efforts and your data dictionary may be doomed from the start.

There are also internal initiatives that can conflict with your project. If the laboratory is planning to install a new chemistry analysis system or getting ready for an inspection, chances are that you won't have their full attention when it comes to getting assistance in defining the laboratory data elements. If an important department is preoccupied with its own project, its active participation is not necessary during the formal project time period. Since the development of a data dictionary is an ongoing process, you can add that department later, as discussed in Chapter 7.

Executive management support
It is crucial for executive management to understand the importance of the project if the data dictionary is to be successful. Executive commitment ensures that the necessary resources will be allocated to the project.

The first level of executive management to recruit is at the Vice President level. The key positions to contact are most likely the Chief Information Officer, Chief Financial Officer, or the Vice President of Support Services. Look for those titles to whom Health Information Management and Information Systems report. They know the value of organized, integrated data. When they are clearly presented with the long-range benefits (accuracy, consistency, quality, no rework, etc.), these administrators will support your project.

Ask one such person to be an administrative sponsor for the project. Sponsorship is not time-consuming, and simply requires a broad understanding of the importance of a data dictionary in the integration of clinical information. Give the sponsor an overview of the scope of the project, the timetable, and the estimated budget. He or she may be able to assist you in finding an IS person to be the database administrator for the software. You will update the sponsor through progress reports so that his or her time commitment is almost nil. The real function the sponsor serves is to champion the project at administrative meetings and ensure that it remains an organizational priority.

The Chief Executive Officer and Board of Directors need to understand the project in the early stages to sanction your efforts. Even if you are simply allowed to give a presentation about the benefits of creating a data dictionary, you must grab their attention and convince them that without the data dictionary, further facility data transfer and interfaces will continue to be inefficient and inaccurate. Well informed executives will buy into the concept of a data dictionary because they know that data is the key to better information. Those aware of the increased demand for information in the marketplace realize that payers, the government, and employers are collecting data and using it to analyze their business. Well-organized internal data has a greater potential to produce quality information that can be presented with confidence to these external parties.

The presentation does not have to be long. You can address key points in 15 minutes. Be ready to address the following issues during the executive presentation:

- State why the project is important to your facility.
- Outline the impetus for the data dictionary.
- Target the presentation to the administrator who controls the allocation of resources.
- Understand the reasons why this project may be questioned and be ready with strong rebuttals for any possible arguments.

Getting time and money committed
In the current cost-cutting environment, getting money committed for any pro-

ject has become difficult. The good news is that unlike committees in which you may have been involved, this is a project; as such it has a discrete beginning, middle, and end. The project is geared toward the design and implementation of a data dictionary where none existed before or to replace several smaller, uncoordinated ones. Once the project team has accomplished its goals, it can disband and the remainder of the work will be to maintain the established data dictionary as an ongoing effort. Maintaining a data dictionary becomes a continuous process of information management.

To get administrative support for the project, you must estimate the cost of the project. Because much of a health care organization's budget is devoted to labor, a valuable and increasingly scarce resource, it will be important to estimate the people you will need and the length of time they will be involved in the project. All of this is covered in depth in Chapter 5.

You also will choose software, as discussed in Chapter 5. You can spend between $300 and $3,000 depending on the type you pick. Compared with the labor expenditure, this is a small fraction of the project's total cost. Budget as much money as possible for software purchases, as it's more difficult to ask for more money later on. You will choose the exact software you need for the database later.

Organizing the team

Why is a team needed? No one person or department can know everything there is to know about the myriad computer systems that generate clinical data. Using a team of people to build the data dictionary not only brings various people's expertise together but it can also cut down the amount of work that one person has to do.

There are two different points of view about setting up teams of people to work on a project of this type. Software developers usually believe that smaller numbers of people are more manageable and able to comply with job assignments and time frames. Wouldn't it be simpler just to have one or two people who are assigned the task of setting up the facility's data dictionary? If the size of your project is very limited in scope, one or two computer systems at most, a smaller team is possible. Consider key members if you limit the size of the group. At a minimum, include representatives from Health Information Management, Information Systems (also known as Data Processing), clinicians (MD and/or RN), ancillary services (lab, radiology, pharmacy), quality improvement, registration areas, financial services, and patient accounts.

The other point of view is that, given the size of a data dictionary project and the scope within the facility, a larger group is needed to understand the complexity and interconnectivity of the systems and to divide up the multitude of responsibilities. You will, most assuredly, spend more time than you want to in meetings and in communicating between meetings. But by using proper meeting control, you can reap the benefits of more people's knowledge; this is critically important in the early planning stages since the data dictionary will eventually cover the entire facility and all of its systems.

Who should be involved?

First and foremost, choose people who have an interest in information. These people will be found in every department and in every corner of the organization. Do not select members based on their level in the organization; instead consider their interest in and enthusiasm for the project and their past performance in following through on project work.

You will look for representatives from any place in the organization that creates, collects, or distributes information. Choose both detail-oriented and big-picture people. Detail-oriented people enjoy learning about how things work together and usually like order, procedures, and structure. They are often interested in figuring out why systems are having problems with the exchange of data. They care about their work, are good producers, and will welcome any enhancement to their productivity, one of the goals of the data dictionary project.

Choose other people who are less detail-oriented but have a big picture understanding of the organization, its structure, and its future goals and objectives.

These people will complement the detail-oriented members—you could have two people from one large department, one providing detail about the department system and the other who understands where the data comes from, how it is used in their department, and where it goes. Something for you to consider: department directors and managers are not necessarily a good choice for team members because they have other responsibilities and new projects will come up that they will consider even more important than the data dictionary project. Use them in an advisory role by adding them to a steering committee that will meet less frequently than the project team. This is discussed later in this chapter in the section on roles and responsibilities.

Where should they be from?
Cross-functional representation is essential in designing a facility-wide data dictionary. Health care facilities are becoming more complex. No type of health care provider is exempt from this increasing complexity; this includes small rural clinics, hospice agencies, metropolitan teaching hospitals, and nationwide health care systems. This complexity is aggravated by all the different types of computer systems with clinical, financial, and administrative data. No one person or department can understand all the intricacies and requirements of the entire system. Multi-departmental representation ensures that all needs will be better addressed.

One way to determine who should participate is to examine the different service areas of your facility and pinpoint the users of electronic data. In a hospital or clinic setting you can divide up the types of computer systems into the following three categories (see Sidebar 3A):

- clinical,
- ancillary services, and
- administrative/support.

The clinical areas may be limited in terms of computerization but their involvement is key since they generate the main product of health care—patient care. Finding physicians or nurses who are interested in computerization is some-

SIDEBAR 3A - Types of Computer Systems

Clinical
 Order Communications/Results
 Nursing
 Physical and Occupational Therapy
 Operating Room System
 Emergency Services

Ancillary services
 Laboratory
 Clinical Pathology
 Radiology
 Pharmacy
 Dietary
 Cardiology
 Dialysis

Administrative/support
 HIM
 Cancer Registry
 Case Mix
 Decision Support
 IS
 Patient Accounts
 Admitting/Registration
 Quality Management
 Contracting/Marketing
 Medical Staff
 Medical Library

times a difficult task. Some of the newer members of the medical or nursing staff may have more time or interest, especially if they had recent computer training in school. Appeal to them by assuring them that the end result will be better patient care and decreased frustration because clinical data will be integrated. If they say that they don't have time, make them advisors, add them to the steering committee, and use them as resources to help solve difficult problems.

The ancillary service areas such as Laboratory, Radiology, and Pharmacy provide diagnostic and therapeutic services for the patients or customers. These areas have had computer systems for years but these systems have often been stand-alone, generating data on paper. They are being interfaced with mainframes or are exchanging data with other systems through interface engines. They are vitally interested in receiving demographic and clinical data, and in sending out their own.

Administrative and support areas include Health Information Management, Admitting or Registration, Patient Accounts, Quality Management, and all the areas that receive clinical information. These areas are the underpinnings of the organization, allowing the clinicians and technicians to perform their duties, receive the data, and generate their own data. Their data also provides the information necessary to keep the health care organization in good shape, from a business perspective.

In Chapter 5, you will define the scope of your project, limit the number of computer systems to start with, and choose a starter set of data elements to define during your project. You may modify your team members once you have decided on these specifics.

Is the representation adequate?

You may discover either in the early stages or along the way that you have omitted an important representative. You may also decide that there are other roles or temporary positions whereby people can be used as resources or advisors to portions of the data dictionary project. The busy clinician is one example. A person who is well qualified but difficult to work with can be placed in a temporary position or asked to perform a specific function where he or she does not need to work with others. If you approach the team building from this point of view, it will be simple to add (or subtract) people as needed.

Political concerns are always an issue. Is there someone in a powerful position who does not want this project to succeed? Are there departments that will be offended by not being asked to participate or give their input? These negative influences can be made positive by adopting a philosophy of inclusion. The bottom line is that this project will contribute to improved patient care by providing useful data and clinical information.

When you are in the early stages of deciding who should participate, obtain input from a wide variety of people from across the organization. Send a simple survey (see Sidebar 3B) throughout the facility which will serve the dual purpose of informing people what the project is about and giving those who have anything to contribute an opportunity to "raise their hands." Not everyone needs to be added to the team but their input can enhance the project by ensuring that important concerns are addressed.

Is there a role for vendors?

Some vendors offer a built-in data dictionary in their system. If the vendor supports a major clinical system and has assigned a local representative to your facility, ask that vendor to attend your meetings. The vendor may have access to expertise that will assist you in your database design and may have been involved in similar projects with other facilities. If the vendor cannot afford the time, ask for the documentation of the vendor's data dictionary. This will be a wonderful starting point for defining the data elements in that particular system.

Roles and responsibilities

Now that you've chosen your team members, it is important to define individual roles and responsibilities. Not only does this clarify the process but it also allows the meetings to progress smoothly and efficiently. Each participant

SIDEBAR 3B - Departmental Survey Form

DATE: _____

TO: _____ DEPARTMENT_____

FROM: _____
      Administrative Sponsor, Data Dictionary Project

_____
      Project Leader, Data Dictionary Project

Our facility is building an organization-wide data dictionary. A data dictionary is an ordered collection of data that describes and locates each data element in an information system. Data dictionaries contribute to uniform data for complete and reliable analysis of patient care and disease trends. The retrieval and use of information is presently limited by inconsistencies in the way that findings, problems, medications, and other data are named.

We are soliciting your input by asking you to respond to the questions below. If you have any questions or would like to discuss the project in greater detail, please contact the project leader at extension _____.

1. Name of your main departmental system containing clinical data.
   _____

2. Names of other departmental systems that contain clinical data.
   _____

3. Systems that download data to your departmental systems. _____
   _____

4. Systems to which your clinical data is uploaded. _____
   _____

5. Known data collection problems with the clinical data elements.
   _____
   _____

SIDEBAR 3B - Departmental Survey Form (continued)

6. Known data use problems with the clinical data elements.
_____
_____

7. Would you be interested in contributing to the data dictionary project?
_____ yes _____ no

8. Describe potential contributions. _____
_____

Thank you for your answers.

Your response is KEY to the data dictionary project's success!

should know what the group as a whole is being asked to do, what the project leader's responsibilities are, and what his or her own individual tasks will be. Specific responsibilities are covered in depth in Chapters 5 and 6. The following are some general comments for your reference.

Generally, the project leader and administrative sponsor will work together to decide on the project scope, schedule, and budget. The database administrator and team members will then be chosen. The leader and database administrator work together to set up the actual database, but the team members are the departmental resources who will assist the group by defining the data elements in their computer systems. The team meets every two weeks, and the steering committee meets periodically with them throughout the project. After the project is finished the departmental team members will continue to participate in the development of the data dictionary by continually adding new data elements to the starter set of data elements.

Administrative sponsor and steering committee

As discussed earlier, having an administrative sponsor ensures that your project remains an organizational priority. The sponsor assists initially in defining project scope and approving a project budget and schedule. He or she will attend the first meeting and will be updated through progress reports.

A steering committee is a core group made up of department directors and managers and key people, like physicians and nurses, who may have little time to devote to the project. The steering committee meets with the team at the beginning, middle, and end of the project. They may also schedule ad hoc meetings to resolve conflicts or problems.

Database administrator

The database administrator will assist the project leader in designing the database, will recommend the appropriate type of database, and will work with the team members to design forms and user views.

Project team members

The project team members will do system research and carry out task assignments. Being a team member has some general responsibilities. A team member must become a participant by expressing his or her views, reservations, and potential problems. Team members can help meetings stay on track by addressing the topic at hand, and staying positive (sometimes against all odds). Good team members realize that effective use of time means enhanced productivity, creative solutions, clearly defined tasks, and meetings that end on time.

Project leader

The project leader has a busy and varied role. Initially the leader will define the project scope, develop a schedule and budget, and oversee meetings. Practical attributes include credibility and a good track record of successful project implementations. You need an understanding of complexity of systems and their interrelationships and a broad-based understanding of the organizational parts and how they relate to the whole. In this project, it is helpful to have a basic understanding of computer systems.

To be an effective team leader, you should have practice in planning techniques and familiarity with monitoring and evaluation skills. As the project leader you must have an understanding of group dynamics. At times, you need to be a team participant, but you must also have strong leadership qualities. These include dedication, the determination to carry the project to its end, internal motivation, and commitment. Along with strong interpersonal and communication skills you should be diplomatic and have the ability to understand and resolve political problems.

If all of this sounds overwhelming, don't worry. If you are well organized and prepared, you can successfully complete the project. We have all been members of committees and felt that we could have run things better. Here is your chance to make a difference. There are several good references provided for you in the Resources section at the end of the book. The other alternative is to use a skilled meeting facilitator. This will give you more time to concentrate on the other responsibilities. Whether you or a facilitator lead the meeting, there are some key principles discussed in the next chapter that will contribute to efficient, effective meetings.

Notes

Chapter 4
Meetings and Communications

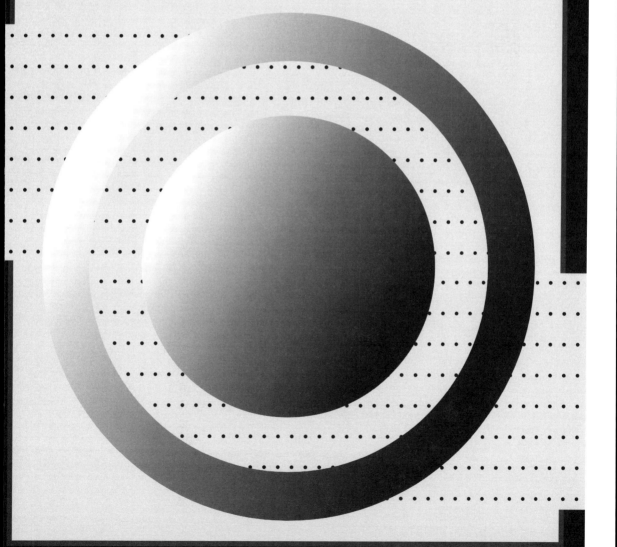

Chapter 4
Meetings and Communications

This chapter covers the team meetings and communications during the life of the data dictionary project. Effective meetings management requires the project leader to have top notch organizational skills during the meetings and to provide clear reports and communication after the meetings.

Meeting organization

Good meetings are well structured and organized. Since you are spending organizational resources every time you convene this group, you want to ensure that time is well spent. To understand the cost of convening a one-hour meeting, multiply the number of people in the meeting by the average hourly wage (include 30% more for benefits). For example, if you are in Ohio in a medium-sized inpatient hospital, and have a range of team members, from some clerical staff to supervisors or technicians, the average hourly cost could be $25.00 per person. If you have 10 people in the room, you are spending $250 every time you meet. If you have 20 people in the meeting, you double the cost. Spend your resources wisely.

One way to efficiently use the team's time is to send out an agenda (see Sidebar 4A) ahead of time so the participants know what topics will be addressed at the meeting. As the project progresses, the agendas will also serve to remind them of their responsibilities and due dates.

The first meeting will be an introductory one to define the project's goal and delineate the process that will be used. Solicit your executive sponsor's support by having him or her give the first call to order, a brief overview of the project and its importance in information management. You then introduce the team members and explain their roles and how responsibilities will be delegated, the project timeline, and how frequently the team will meet. Lastly, you will schedule the next meeting and adjourn.

Chapter 4

SIDEBAR 4A - Agenda—Data Dictionary Project	
Meeting #1	
1. Call to order	Executive sponsor
2. Introduction of members	All
3. Review of goals	Project leader
4. Review of committee process	Project leader
5. Roles and responsibilities	Project leader
6. Upcoming schedule/timeline	Project leader
7. Potential obstacles	All
8. Other business	All
9. Meeting assessment and critique	All
10. Schedule next meeting	All
11. Adjourn meeting	Project leader

Another meeting management tip is to start and end the meeting on time. Agree that those who are late will be responsible for finding out what they missed. Keep the meetings on track by dealing with one issue at a time. As project leader, you will have to control those members who get off track.

A good team fosters participation from everyone in the group and both the leader and the participants should encourage quiet people to express their views or reservations. You can engender creative solutions by encouraging brainstorming, a method of problem solving whereby members of a group spontaneously contribute ideas that are not initially judged. The rules are that no idea is a bad idea and that everything is potentially a good idea or at least a neutral one.

Documentation

Good documentation is an essential component of any project. Documentation clarifies understanding and records data and decisions for the database administrator and team leader. This documentation can later be used as the basis of further work and serve as a means of answering future questions like "Why was it done this way?" A data dictionary project, by its own nature, requires very precise documentation because the data dictionary is metadata—data about data.

Your meeting documentation will help you to evaluate if your meeting objectives were met. When you can demonstrate that the meeting objectives were met, you show progress toward the goal and the team members will feel that their time is being well spent. The documentation will record what happened, what decisions were made, what problems were solved, what problems still remain, and what the team members are doing. As team leader, you will clearly see if you are getting the results you expected and can make adjustments to the process if you are not.

There are a variety of ways that you can document committee activities, assign responsibilities, and record committee accomplishments. Taking minutes is one type of recordkeeping activity. The negative side to this is that someone has to take minutes and type them up later. There are simpler alternatives to minutes, alternatives that will make the process seem less formidable, including flip charts and process lists.

Flip charts
Use flip charts on large easels to record main points and key ideas. Use a separate sheet to record anything else that causes lengthy discussion or strong contention. When a point is noted, members feel as though recording it

allows them to move on to the next point. The leader and members are jointly responsible to ensure their points are recorded when they feel strongly about them. At the end of the meeting, date these sheets and retain them as a meeting history.

Process list

A process list is another way to record committee activities (see Table 4A). Brief notes are taken in a word processor table in columnar format. Identify the topic, summarize the discussion and recommendations, assign any tasks to the responsible member, and give the time frame for completion. Not only is this method easy, it is simple to review. If documentation goes to the steering committee or project sponsor, they can skim the topic column to get an overview and focus on anything they want to know more about. Team members use the process list to ensure that they have completed all of their assignments on time. The team leader uses it to monitor activities and to set a starting point for the next meeting. When you reconvene, use the previous process list, update it by adding new items and deleting completed ones, and save it as a new document.

Progress reports

Progress reports are an excellent way to summarize activity during a project. Good progress reporting helps foster communication throughout the project between team members, the administrative sponsor, the steering committee, and the team leader. These reports can also capture historical data as a byproduct that can be referenced for future project management success. Progress reports are as simple as filling in the blanks in the following categories:

- Executive summary/overview
- Schedule status
- Accomplishments/tasks finished
- Planned work
- Project analysis
- Additional detail

TABLE 4A - Process List—Data Dictionary Project 07-17-97

Present: K. Caldwell, Lab, J. Lewis, Radiology, G. Croy, Registration, D. Chase, Nursing, S. Wong, IS, J. Smith, Pharmacy, J. Muniz, HIM, L. Elder, Finance, T. Young, Decision Support, M. Dietzel, Administration

Topic	Discussion	Recommendation	Responsibility	Due Date
DD project goals	DD project overview and goals presented by M. Dietzel	N/A	N/A	N/A
Committee process	T. Young gave overview of committee process	N/A	N/A	N/A
Roles and responsibilities	T. Young reviewed R & Rs of all team members	N/A	N/A	N/A
Upcoming schedule	T. Young distributed schedule of activities (attached)	N/A	All	As scheduled

TABLE 4A - Process List—Data Dictionary Project 07-17-97 (continued)

Topic	Discussion	Recommendation	Responsibility	Due Date
Potential obstacles	Group discussed 2 conflicting projects - lab will be installing a new chemistry analyzer and radiology will implement a new bar coding system	Lab will work on DD early in project time frame and may drop out of 2 meetings Radiology will discuss impact of bar coding install on DD project and assign new rep. by next meeting	K. Caldwell to meet with S. Wong to begin lab portion J. Lewis to discuss with dept. head	07/24/97 07/31/97
Meeting assessment and critique	Members felt that too much time was spent on materials they could read ahead of time	Leader to prepare pre-work and distribute to team members; team members to review before meeting	T. Young and all	07/28/97
Next meeting	Meetings to be regularly scheduled, every other Friday	Mark calendars	All	N/A

See Table 4B for format and section content suggestions.

Communication

Communication is simply the exchange of information. Whether this takes place orally, in writing, or visually, it is essential that the data dictionary project work be communicated throughout the organization since standardization of data is critical to the organization's success. The project leader is the person responsible for coordinating the project communications. He or she is the recipient of information and can disseminate it upward, downward, and laterally throughout the organization. A successful project encourages and obtains input from all levels.

Audience

There are various audiences for the exchange of information. Within the project team itself, the members initially want to know the background for the project and their roles and responsibilities. They will want updates on the project's status and will contribute information about their departments and computer systems. The regular team meetings ensure that the members give and receive information they need to proceed with their next assignments.

The steering committee and administrative sponsor are interested in receiving regular summary information in the form of project reports. This will keep them informed of progress; this summary can be communicated to administrators and other key people within the organization.

Organizational communications should give general information about the project and focus on how a data dictionary can ensure uniform data collection and alleviate problems that plague the work environment, such as redundant data entry when two systems are unable to exchange information correctly. It is true in every organization, and with any project, that it is vital to keep your sponsors and top management informed of your project status. This includes project delays as well as accomplishments. Don't let your project sponsor or organization management be "surprised" by hearing project news, either good or bad, through the grapevine.

TABLE 4B - Project Report

_____(Project leader name)
_____(Report date)
_____(Time period covered)

EXECUTIVE SUMMARY/OVERVIEW

Brief paragraph or 5–7 bullet points

Project objective

Team purpose

_____
_____
_____
_____
_____

SCHEDULE STATUS

Graphic, (eg, Gantt chart) showing planned and actual dates

_____
_____
_____
_____
_____

ACCOMPLISHMENTS/TASKS FINISHED

Milestones reached

Changes in project

_____
_____
_____
_____
_____

TABLE 4B - Project Report (continued)

PLANNED WORK
General discussion of upcoming tasks

Tasks scheduled but not finished

_____
_____
_____
_____
_____

PROJECT ANALYSIS
Problems and corrective actions

New issues to be dealt with

Changes to project and rationale

Unresolved issues, responsible party, and due date for resolution

_____
_____
_____
_____
_____

ADDITIONAL DETAIL
Any additional detail that the audience may want

Can include screen shots, tables, etc.

_____
_____
_____
_____
_____

Communication techniques

The most effective format for communication depends on the type of audience. For the best results, you need to get the right information to the right people at the right time. This takes thought and careful planning. Try different ways and different levels of detail. Table 4C will help you choose some appropriate communication methods.

With a firm grasp of general meeting and communication skills, you are now ready to tackle the specifics of the project—the planning and design of the data dictionary.

TABLE 4C - Communication Methods		
AUDIENCE	**VERBAL**	**WRITTEN**
Sponsor/Top Management	Presentation Final wrap-up presentation	Regular progress reports Graphical displays Final progress report
Department Managers	Periodic project meetings Voice mail reports	Progress reports Minutes Newsletters
Department Users	One-on-one	Minutes Newsletters E-mail

Chapter 5

Planning and Designing the Data Dictionary

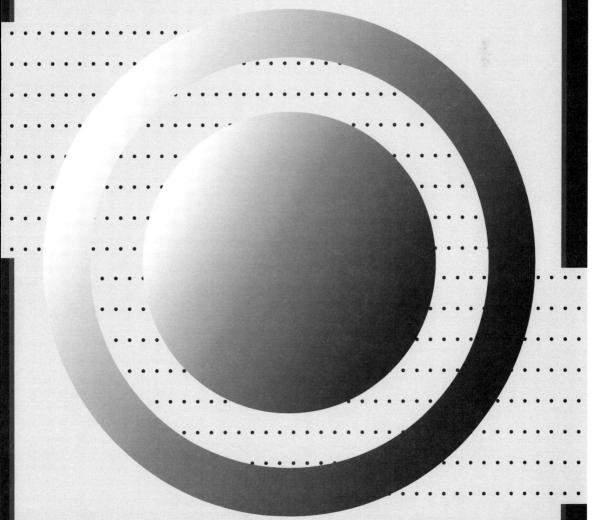

Chapter 5
Planning and Designing the Data Dictionary

Now let's get down to the business of beginning the data dictionary. Beginning is the operative word here because health care organizations have many computer systems and a multitude of databases, so building a comprehensive data dictionary can take several years. In reality, a data dictionary project is never finished.

When you think about the sheer size of it, a data dictionary project can be overwhelming and discouraging. A better approach, both psychologically and procedurally, is to consider this project an organizational commitment to information management (see case study in Chapter 8). The organization must be committed to the ongoing management of information; the development and maintenance of a data dictionary is an important component in this process. It's like weight loss—everyone wants to do it overnight but what it really requires is a lifestyle change. Likewise, a comprehensive data dictionary project cannot be accomplished in a short period of time and it does require an organizational lifestyle change.

Chapters 5 and 6 describe a unique approach to the design and implementation of a data dictionary for a health care facility. They outline a project of realistic size, the development of a data dictionary model and the definition of a set of vital data elements. Too many health care organizations have started out with the best of intentions, to define every important data element in the place. This task is too overwhelming and their good intentions fizzle and fade. What they have left is a partially completed data dictionary that is never used by anyone, except possibly the IS folks.

Our data dictionary project can be accomplished within a three-month period. By agreeing on a limited number of systems and a small set of data elements for the project, the organization is not overwhelmed; it can not only commit to the project but it can complete it. You will design a data dictionary and begin to implement it. Chapter 7 outlines a plan to maintain and expand it over the years.

Define scope of the project

Because the ultimate goal of a data dictionary is to define all data elements, establishing a comprehensive data dictionary will take years. Start with a portion of data definitions that will be valuable to your organization. By beginning with key data your project remains tightly defined and can be completed in a reasonable time frame. Your success will provide momentum for ongoing additions that will eventually build a comprehensive, organization-wide data dictionary.

Limit the number of computer systems

To make the project manageable, you not only have to limit the number of data elements but you also have to limit the number of application systems. If you work at a large facility or health care system, limit the project to four to six departmental systems. Include departments that are very visible and important to the organization's functioning. Success in key departments is valuable to the organization. Smaller, single focus health care organizations, like home health or rehab, should define core elements for all their systems. Likewise, if you have limited time or personnel to devote to this project, you can further limit the number of data elements and systems.

Use a relational database

By using a relational database to build the data dictionary, an organization can take into account the discrepancies in the names and contents of similar data elements in each department and can begin to relate these to national standards. This keeps the structure and entry of the data elements simple, and unstructured ad hoc queries of the data dictionary are possible.

For example, each departmental system (eg, nursing, lab, radiology, billing) has its own data definition for a field, but the users of the data dictionary can do a query on ASTM number 01001, PATIENT NAME, and see a list of data elements from all other computer systems which contain this field. These other systems may call this field NAME, SUBSCRIBER NAME, FULL NAME, or CUSTOMER NAME. Although the name, formats, edits, etc., of the data element differ between systems, the intent of the field is the same: to identify the name of the person receiving health care services. This is similar to a standard dictionary whereby a word has a first or preferred definition and alternate definitions that follow. These alternate definitions are analogous to the departmental system data definitions.

By establishing one core set of MPI data elements and relating these through the ASTM number to other similar data elements in departmental systems, an organization can begin to organize its data definitions, but still allow for the variations in computer systems. The different departments may find participation in this type of data dictionary project more palatable, because they do not have to give up their own definitions, they simply have to relate them to the core dictionary.

Remember, this is a starting point for a comprehensive data dictionary. During the ongoing development and maintenance period, you will add more data elements and more systems. Our project in Chapters 5 and 6 starts with eight departmental systems:

- Clinical systems
    - nursing
    - laboratory
    - radiology
    - pharmacy
- Support systems
    - registration
    - health information (medical records)
    - patient billing
    - decision support

Limit the number of data elements

In the same way that you must limit the number of departmental computer systems, you must also limit the number of data elements. The choice of data elements in this project is based on the concept of patient identification. Patient identification allows health care providers to identify the person receiving the treatment or services.

Patient identification data elements

Patient identification data include common elements such as the patient's name, medical record number, date of birth, sex, and address. This minimal set is commonly called the Master Patient Index (MPI). Additional patient identification data elements include previous names (through marriage, divorce, adoption), aliases, social security number, race, ethnicity, marital status, and occupation. There are many more patient identification data elements that are also used to establish who is responsible for paying the bill (guarantor information) and how it will be paid (insurance information). In assessing data in various computer systems, you find that these same MPI data elements are located in computer systems throughout the organization (see Figure 5A).

Each computer system stores at least one of these data elements (medical record number), and probably more (name, date of birth, sex, address, and phone number). This should be no surprise because every system needs to attribute the data it collects to the correct patient. For example, a pharmacy system receives an order for a medication, either verbally, on paper, or through computer transfer. The pharmacist locates previous prescriptions for that specific patient in the pharmacy system. The order is then filled and documented in the computer system. The same process occurs in a clinic laboratory system, in a radiology practice, or in a hospital nursing system. All of these clinical settings, through their computer systems, must be able to locate previously treated patients, access their records, and document the current treatment.

When data elements are loosely defined there are problems with patient iden-

Planning and Designing the Data Dictionary

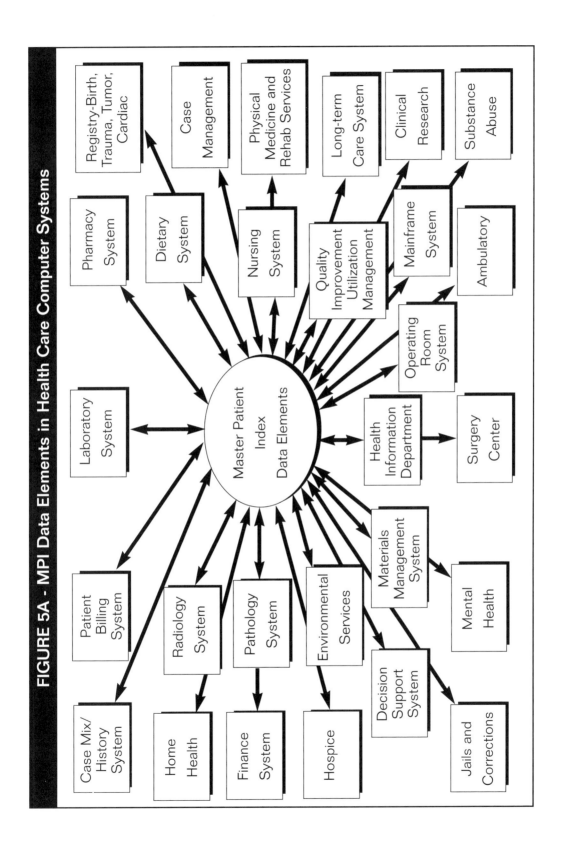

FIGURE 5A - MPI Data Elements in Health Care Computer Systems

tification. For example, one computer system may ignore the hyphen in a last name (Smith-Jenkins) while another computer system may treat it as a separate character. When a registrar searches the ADT system and cannot locate a previous registration, he or she assigns a new medical record number and creates what is commonly known as a duplicate medical record. Now one patient has two separate registrations and two separate medical records. The patient's previous medical history is no longer accessible to the clinicians under a single medical record. Previously known medication allergies that are documented in the first medical record are unknown in the second medical record. The patient care consequences are obvious.

This problem has plagued the paper-based world for years but is becoming more pronounced as facilities combine services or merge with other organizations. Most estimates place the duplicate medical record rate at 5–10% in an average health care facility. In a moderately sized organization containing 500,000 medical record numbers, even with an exceptionally clean MPI, a 2% duplicate rate translates into 10,000 patients whose records cannot be linked together.

The MPI data elements are the key to linking all medical records. Defining the MPI data elements will assist the facility in standardizing usage of this important set of data throughout the organization. By documenting the format of the individual data elements, the departments will understand the rules of use for each data element. This will reduce the inconsistencies in the computer systems and therefore dramatically decrease the creation of duplicate medical records.

A data dictionary starter set
Since correct patient identification is the key to the linking of medical records of one patient throughout a health care system and the MPI data elements are common to every computer system in the organization, these data elements are a good starting point for the data dictionary project. The integrity of these data elements affects all computer systems in the organization, except possibly purely administrative systems such as human resources and

engineering. Defining the MPI data also allows an organization to focus on an important set of data elements that are a core building block for the computerized patient record (CPR).

Use of ASTM standards
The MPI data set is well defined in the American Society of Testing and Materials (ASTM) E 1384-96 "Standard Guide of Content and Structure of the Computer-Based Patient Record." This standard guide was issued in 1996 to promote consistent and efficient data transfer. The guide identifies the content and logical structure of a CPR and defines the relationship of data coming from diverse application systems. The standard promulgates a common vocabulary for the content of a CPR and outlines data items common in the paper medical record. This standard is available at a nominal charge from the ASTM. The address is listed in the Resources section at the end of this book.

Table 5A lists 26 data elements from the ASTM guide that are common patient identification fields in many computer systems. The columns list the ASTM number, the data element name (or "field name"), the short name (or "field code"), and a brief description of the data element. These data elements and many more are located in the ASTM standard guide in Annex A1 "CPR Data Dictionary Resource."

By following the ASTM E 1384-96 national standards for naming the MPI data elements, an organization will have the foundation for standardization across computer systems throughout the organization and eventually allow the linkage or exchange of data with external organizations and agencies. A health care organization should strive to use standard definitions and insist that current and prospective vendors incorporate these standards into their software. By doing so, an organization can begin to reconcile some of the discrepancies in data definitions and the impact these discrepancies have on the facility.

Develop a project schedule
Because this project is broken down into a limited number of data elements and departmental systems, it can be finished within a 12-week period. During

Chapter 5

\multicolumn{4}{c|}{TABLE 5A - ASTM Data Elements}			
ASTM E 1344 Number	**Field Name**	**Field Code**	**Description**
01001	PATIENT NAME	PersName	Person receiving health care services and about whom records containing data about those services are collected
01002	PREVIOUSLY REGISTERED NAME	PersPrevRegName	A last name changed due to marriage or initiated by patient; a former name; a maiden name
01010	ALIAS	PersAliasName	A name added to, or substituted for, the proper name of a person; an assumed name
01015	PATIENT NO.	PtIDNum	Unique number assigned by the provider to: 1) distinguish the patient and his/her medical record from all others in the institution, 2) facilitate retrieval of the record, and 3) facilitate posting of payment

TABLE 5A - ASTM Data Elements (continued)			
ASTM E 1344 Number	**Field Name**	**Field Code**	**Description**
01016	UNIVERSAL PATIENT HEALTH NO.	PtUniversalHealth Num	Permanent, unique number used by all providers and third party payers in conjunction with establishing and using the longitudinal record. It will link services for the individual across care systems.
01020	SSAN	PersSSANCode SocialSecurity AcctNum	A pseudo social security number may be assigned if patient does not have a SSAN.
01025	ARCHIVE DATA	PtRecordArchive LocName	The locations of linked fragmented records; it also identifies permanent storage locations of inactive archived records.
01027	RECORD-HOLDING LOCATION ID	PtRecHold LocationID	Code identifier of a health care site that maintains a primary record of care about this patient.

Chapter 5

TABLE 5A - ASTM Data Elements (continued)			
ASTM E 1344 Number	**Field Name**	**Field Code**	**Description**
01030	LOCATION OF CHART	PtPaperChart LocName	Location of the paper chart or the location of automated MR (medical record)
01032	DATE-TIME OF BIRTH	PersBirthDtm	The exact time of the birth event; age is generated from the DOB if needed; time can be included for newborns.
01040	SEX	PersGenderCode (As recorded at the start of care)	Distinction of gender
01042	RACE	PersRaceCode	The major biologic Class to which the patient belongs as a result of a pedigree analysis or with which the patient identifies him/herself in cases where the data are not conclusive.

TABLE 5A - ASTM Data Elements (continued)

ASTM E 1344 Number	Field Name	Field Code	Description
01045	ETHNIC GROUP	PtEthnicGroup Code	That cultural group with which the patient identifies him/herself either by means of recorded family data or personal preference. A patient may belong to several such groups depending upon heritage, language, nationality, or social association.
01052	MARITAL STATUS	PersMaritalStatus Code	Marital status of the patient at the start of care. NEVER MARRIED includes annulment of only marriage. SEPARATED: married persons living apart except institutionalized. WIDOWED: spouse died and not remarried. DIVORCED: legally divorced and not remarried.

TABLE 5A - ASTM Data Elements (continued)

ASTM E 1344 Number	Field Name	Field Code	Description
01057	PATIENT'S LANGUAGE	PtLanguageCode	A term indicating the language most frequently spoken by the patient in communicating with health care practitioners; if more than one language is spoken, record the frequency with which each one is used in the health care setting.
01065	OCCUPATION	OccOccupationName	The employment, business, or a course of action in which the patient is engaged (eg, "student").
01075	PRESENT EMPLOYER NAME	EmplrPresentEmployerName	Name of workplace (organization) or employer's full name. That part providing a position (and compensation) for an employee.
01090	FAMILY MEMBER NAME	FAMMbrName	The name of each family member.

TABLE 5A - ASTM Data Elements (continued)

ASTM E 1344 Number	Field Name	Field Code	Description
01090.11	FAMILY MEMBER FEMALE PARENT MAIDEN NAME	FAMMbrFemaleParentName	The name of the biologic female parent of the patient to be used for family pedigrees. It is the full name of a newborn infant's mother.
01095	PATIENT PERMANENT ADDRESS	PersPermanentAddressText	The usual residence and/or address of the patient as defined by the payer organization. May be referred to as the "Mailing Address."
01096	PATIENT PRIOR ADDRESS	PtPriorAddressText	Address prior to the current one at which the patient resided.
01100	HOME PHONE	PersHomePhoneNum	The phone numbers of both permanent and temporary addresses.
01110	EMERG. CONT. (REL/FR.)	PtEmergContName	Person to be notified in case of emergency, if needed.

| TABLE 5A - ASTM Data Elements (continued) ||||
ASTM E 1344 Number	Field Name	Field Code	Description
01112	EMERG. CONT. RELAT.	PtEmergCont RelationCode	A code denoting the relationship of the emergency contact to the patient.
01115	EMERG. CONT. ADDRESS	PtEmergCont AddressText	The address of the person to contact in any emergency situation.
01117	EMERG. CONT. H. PHONE	PtEmergCont HPhoneNum	The most appropriate phone number of the emergency contact person.

Adapted from Annex A1; CPR data dictionary resource. In: Standard Guide of Content and Structure of the Computer-based Patient Record. American Society of Testing and Materials, 1996.

this time, the project leader devotes eight hours a week, the database administrator spends 20 hours a week, and the eight departmental team members spend a decreasing amount of time on the project during the 12-week period. The steering committee spends a total of only three hours per person. Table 5B shows the various representatives in the first column. The subsequent columns indicate the week of the project. Each row details the amount of hours a representative will spend on particular weeks of the project. The right-hand column totals the hours for each representative. This project will take a grand total of 718 hours.

The project timeline is agreed upon by the administrative champion and the project leader. The project leader sets the project start date, the project com-

TABLE 5B - Project Team Labor Budget In Hours Per Week

TEAM MEMBER	WEEK													TOTAL HOURS
	0	1	2	3	4	5	6	7	8	9	10	11	12	
Project Leader	3	8	8	8	8	8	8	8	8	8	8	8	8	99
Administrative Sponsor	3													3
Database Administrator		20	20	20	20	20	20	20	20	20	20	20	20	240
8 Department Directors		8				8							8	24
Laboratory			8	8	8	4	4	2	2	2	2	2	2	44
Radiology			8	8	8	4	4	2	2	2	2	2	2	44
Nursing			8	8	8	4	4	2	2	2	2	2	2	44
Pharmacy			8	8	8	4	4	2	2	2	2	2	2	44
Registration			8	8	8	4	4	2	2	2	2	2	2	44
HIM			8	8	8	4	4	2	2	2	2	2	2	44
Finance			8	8	8	4	4	2	2	2	2	2	2	44
Decision Support			8	8	8	4	4	2	2	2	2	2	2	44
TOTAL PROJECT HOURS														**718**

pletion date, a list of tasks, and the order in which they are accomplished. The project leader also estimates the number of personnel required to accomplish the tasks, and the skill level necessary to perform the tasks.

A project schedule is built on the experience of the team leader, the information available at the time of planning, and good guesswork. As in any planning process, unforeseen circumstances or external problems can arise at any point in the project. A project planning tool such as a Gantt-type matrix can assist the project leader in developing the timeline and in communicating to the administrative sponsor, steering committee and team members. A Gantt chart shows project progress in relation to time; it also serves as a useful tracking tool to keep the project on schedule. A Gantt chart is shown in Table 5C with the tasks and time frames outlined.

Develop a project budget
The methodology of developing a data dictionary around a limited set of data elements allows the project to be affordable. In this example, the project has a span of 12 weeks. Nine administrative employees give a total of three hours each to the project. Ten employees are participating at varying degrees of involvement. The total number of hours allotted to the project are 718, or 18 person weeks. This project costs approximately $18,450 in total. This cost includes $17,950 in direct personnel costs and $500 if the facility needs to purchase database software for the data dictionary database. This figure averages the hourly rate of pay at $25.00 per hour and does not include any benefits (health care, holiday, long-term disability, etc.) or additional payroll costs. If your facility wants a more accurate estimate, multiply each member's salary level (translated into hourly rates) by a benefits factor (usually 30–35%) to get a more exact figure.

Additional costs for this project are minimal. Project management and project support are built in, and there are no travel costs, unless you want to do a site visit to see a successful data dictionary in action. Alternatively, input from peers can be obtained in a telephone interview. The only space cost is for a meeting room for three meetings for 10 people and another three meetings for

TABLE 5C - Gantt Chart

TASK	WEEK NUMBER												
	0	1	2	3	4	5	6	7	8	9	10	11	12
Initial set-up work													
Select project manager and database administrator	X												
Define project scope	X												
Define tasks and responsibilities	X												
Develop project schedule	X												
Develop project budget	X												
Select steering committee and project team	X												
Meeting #1 Kick-off		X											
With administrative sponsor													
Steering Committee													
Project team													
Departmental system analysis		X	X	X									
Design database specifications		X	X	X									
Meeting #2													
With project team				X	X								
Review departmental data				X									
Review ASTM standards													
Feedback to department managers					X								
Define core data elements					X								

TABLE 5C - Gantt Chart (continued)

TASK	\multicolumn{13}{c}{WEEK NUMBER}												
	0	1	2	3	4	5	6	7	8	9	10	11	12
Meeting #3						X							
With steering committee													
Project team													
Review department feedback						X							
Incorporate changes							X						
Select and order DD database							X						
Progress report to administrative sponsor							X						
Meeting #4								X					
With project team													
Design user views									X				
Finalize data entry									X				
Meeting #5										X			
With project team													
Train all users											X		
Meeting #6 Wrap-up												X	
With steering committee													
Project team													
Final report to administrator sponsor													X

18 people. Training time and costs are included in the project itself. The participants will be trained on the use of the database during the implementation phase. The software costs are minimal. If the facility does not currently have a preferred database software, excellent database software costs between $200 and $500. Since the database can be developed on an existing desktop computer, there are no hardware costs.

Industry studies on the implementation of the CPR have set the price per hospital in a range from $2 million for a medium-sized facility to $40 million for a larger facility. Clearly, the establishment of a data dictionary is one of the least expensive tasks of CPR preparation.

Design

The next stage in planning this project is design; this is a creative process and for the data dictionary project includes defining the tables of the data dictionary database, analyzing the departmental systems, outlining the database system requirements, and selecting the appropriate software.

Database design

Using the MPI data elements and the ASTM E 1384-96 standards, the data dictionary in this example is made up of nine database tables, or "files." There is a "core" table that uses ASTM E 1384-96 standards, and eight departmental tables that have the ASTM number as the primary key (see Figure 5B).

Core file data elements
Table 5D lists 10 critical MPI data elements for this book's example. We chose these 10 as the core data elements for the project because they are found in many computer systems and assist registrars in clearly establishing a patient's identification. The core table will use the ASTM number, field name, field code, and description exactly as they appear in the E 1384-96 standard guide. These data definitions will be used by the health care facility as standards to which all other like data elements in all the computer systems throughout the health care organization will be "related" (see Figure 5B).

Chapter 5

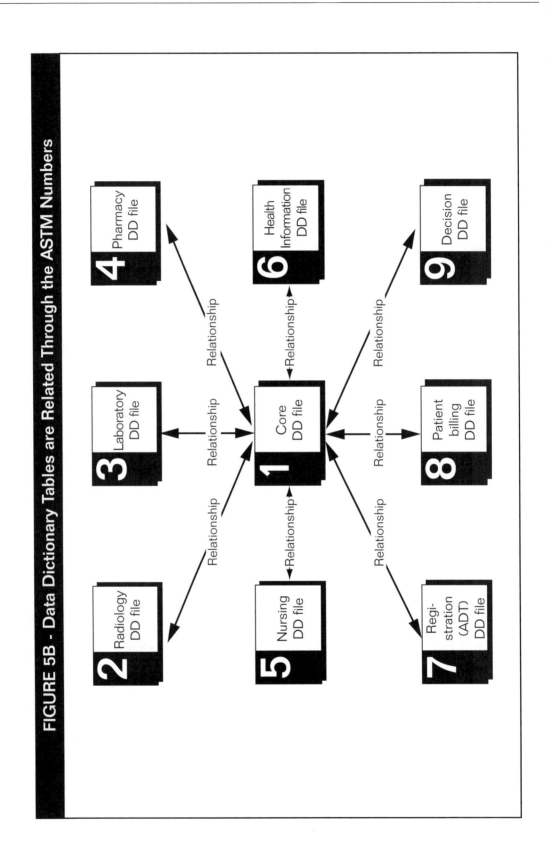

FIGURE 5B - Data Dictionary Tables are Related Through the ASTM Numbers

Planning and Designing the Data Dictionary

TABLE 5D - MPI Data Elements		
ASTM NUMBER	**FIELD NAME**	**FIELD CODE**
01001	PATIENT NAME	PersName
01002	PREVIOUSLY REGISTERED NAME	PersPrevRegName
01015	PATIENT NO.	PtIDNum
01020	SSAN	PersSSANCodeSocialSecurityAcctNum
01032	DATE-TIME OF BIRTH	PersBirthDtm
01040	SEX	PersGenderCode
01065	OCCUPATION	OccOccupationName
01090.11	FAMILY MEMBER FEMALE PARENT MAIDEN NAME	FAMMbrFemaleParentName
01095	PATIENT PERMANENT ADDRESS	PersPermanentAddressText
01100	HOME PHONE	PersHomePhoneNum

In other words, if a radiology clerk interviews a patient and enters this set of 10 data elements into the radiology system, they will locate any previous registrations for that patient. These 10 data elements are not the only ones that can be used in your core table; your facility may choose to add or subtract data elements. Remember, for your initial project, keep the list short and manageable.

Data dictionary files
It is important that each of the 10 core data elements be defined fully and that certain "attributes" are described. The attributes to be defined include ASTM Number, Field Name, Synonyms, and several others. Attributes document characteristics for each data element, such as the length of the field or whether it is alpha or numeric. Table 5E shows the Registration (ADT) system database file

TABLE 5E - Data Dictionary Attributes for Patient Name

Attribute Name	Attribute Description	Example
ASTM NUMBER	Database key number that uniquely identifies this data element	01001
FIELD NAME	Name of the data element	PATIENT NAME
FIELD CODE	Abbreviated field name used by the computer software to textually identify this field	PersName
DESCRIPTION	Simple description of this data element	Person receiving health care services and about whom records containing data about those services are collected
SYNONYMS	Other names by which data element is known	Full name, legal name
SOURCE	Personnel or system originating data	ADT system in registration areas
FORMAT TYPE	Alpha, numeric, combination, integer, decimal, character, date or logical (yes/no, true/false, etc.)	alpha
LEXICON USED	Text, ICD, CPT, DSM4	text
LENGTH	Number of characters in the field	33
ALLOWABLE RANGE	Defines the limits within which the values for this field are considered valid	N/A

TABLE 5E - Data Dictionary Attributes for Patient Name (continued)		
Attribute Name	**Attribute Description**	**Example**
CONFIDENTIALITY LEVEL	Facility defined, degree to which the contents of this field are confidential	Level 2
ACCESS LEVEL	Facility defined, the password level necessary to access this field	Level 2
EDITS	Enforces data entry according to rules such as mandatory completion, record counts, check digits, code verification tables, valid field combinations	No punctuation, symbols, numbers
RESPONSIBILITY	Department or employee responsible for verifying that data is valid and input correctly	Registration and Health Information
UPDATE AUTHORITY	Type of user who can modify this data element	Health Information
FINAL AUTHORITY	Type of user who has the final authority on what is entered in this field	Health Information

with 16 attributes that describe the data element PATIENT NAME. The first column describes the field attribute. The second column contains a brief description of the attribute and the third column gives an example for the data element PATIENT NAME.

When the data dictionary database is set up in column and row format, the columns and rows are switched from the example in Table 5E. The ADT file

Chapter 5

TABLE 5F - Data Dictionary Database File

ASTM No.	Field name	Field code	Description	Synonyms	Source
01001	PATIENT NAME	PersName	Person receiving health....	Full name, legal name	ADT System
01002	PREVIOUSLY REGISTERED NAME	PersPrevRegName	A last name changed....	Former name, alias	ADT System
01015	PATIENT NO.	PtIDNum	Unique number assigned...	Medical record number	ADT System
01020	SSAN	PersSSANCode SocialSecurity AcctNum	A pseudo social security...	Social Security Number	ADT System
01032	DATE-TIME OF BIRTH	PersBirthDtm	The exact time of the birth...	DOB	ADT System
01040	SEX	PersGenderCode	Distinction of gender.	Gender	ADT System
01065	OCCUPATION	OccOccupationName	The employment, business....	Profession	ADT System
01090.11	FAMILY MEMBER FEMALE PARENT MAIDEN NAME	FAMMbrFemaleParentName	The name of the biologic...	Mother's maiden name	ADT System
01095	PATIENT PERMANENT ADDRESS	PersPermanentAddressTest	The usual residence and...	Home address	ADT System
01100	HOME PHONE	PersHomePhoneNum	The phone numbers of...	Telephone number	ADT System

12 Weeks to a Successful Data Dictionary

TABLE 5F - Data Dictionary Database File (continued)

ASTM No.	Format type	Lexicon	Length	Range	Confident.	Access	Edits	Responsibility	Update Authority	Final Authority
01001	Alpha	Text	33	N/A	Level 2	Level 2	No punctuation, symbols or numbers	REG/HIM	REG/HIM	REG
01002	Alpha	Text	33	N/A	Level 2	Level 2	No punctuation, symbols or numbers	REG/HIM	REG/HIM	REG
01015	Numeric	N/A	11	N/A	Level 2	Level 2	N/A	HIM	REG/HIM	HIM
01020	Numeric	N/A	9	N/A	Level 2	Level 2	N/A	REG	REG/HIM	PAA
01032	Date	N/A	12	N/A	Level 2	Level 2	Date cannot be after admission date	REG/HIM	REG/HIM	HIM
01040	Numeric	N/A	1	1-5	Level 2	Level 2	No numbers allowed outside of range	HIM	REG/HIM	HIM
01065	Alpha	N/A	25	N/A	Level 2	Level 2	N/A	REG	REG/HIM	PAA
01090.11	Alpha	Text	20	N/A	Level 2	Level 2	No punctuation, symbols or numbers	REG	REG/HIM	PAA
01095	Combination	N/A	45	N/A	Level 2	Level 2	N/A	REG	REG/HIM	PAA
01100	Numeric	N/A	13	N/A	Level 2	Level 2	N/A	REG	REG/HIM	PAA

FIGURE 5C - Departmental Survey Form

DATE: _____

TO: _____ DEPARTMENT _____

FROM: _____ Administrative Sponsor,
Data Dictionary Project

_____ Project Leader, Data Dictionary Project

Your department has been chosen as a key department to participate in the Data Dictionary Project. The initial steps in developing a data dictionary include a survey of your departmental system(s) and 10 key patient identification data elements. If you need any assistance, please contact the project leader at extension _____.

1. Name of the main departmental system containing MPI data
   _____

2. Names of other departmental systems that contain MPI data
   _____

3. Titles of employee(s) responsible for collecting the MPI data
   _____

4. Systems that download MPI data
   _____

5. Systems to which MPI data is uploaded
   _____

6. Known data collection problems with the MPI data elements
   _____
   _____
   _____
   _____

> **FIGURE 5C - Departmental Survey Form (continued)**
>
> 7. Known data use problems with the MPI data elements
>
>   _____
>   _____
>   _____
>   _____
>
> For each departmental system in 1 and 2, please fill out a separate "Departmental Data Dictionary File Contents" form for each of the 10 data elements.
>
> **Thank you for your answers.**
>
> **Your participation is KEY to the data dictionary project's success!**

would look like Table 5F; the columns show the attributes and the rows are the various data elements. Notice that each data element uses the ASTM number as the primary key. This allows each of the departmental files to be related to the core file and all of the other departmental system files.

Departmental system data elements
Each departmental table is set up with the ASTM number as the primary key (see Figure 5B). The field name and field code from ASTM E 1384-96 are also used. The team members use surveys and interviews to gather the necessary information about each one of the data elements in their own departmental system. The project leader and the database administrator are responsible for developing a Departmental Survey Form (see Figure 5C). This survey form provides helpful background information on each of the departments participating in the project. Questions 4 and 5 allow the project leader and database administrator to understand the relationships between computer systems. Questions

TABLE 5G - Departmental Data Dictionary File Contents

Note: Departmental representative to fill out one form for each key data element in computer system

Attribute Name	Attribute Description
ASTM NUMBER	
FIELD NAME	
FIELD CODE	
DESCRIPTION	
SYNONYMS	
SOURCE	
FORMAT TYPE	
LEXICON USED	
LENGTH	
ALLOWABLE RANGE	
CONFIDENTIALITY LEVEL	
ACCESS LEVEL	
EDITS	
RESPONSIBILITY	
UPDATE AUTHORITY	
FINAL AUTHORITY	

6 and 7 may reveal unknown data collection, transmission, and usage problems. Although these problems will not be addressed during the data dictionary project, they should be documented. There is a good chance that some of the problems will be alleviated through the standardization of data definitions.

Hand these surveys out to the project team members at the kick-off meeting. Each departmental team member is responsible for getting the survey completed and to do this effectively, he or she will need to interview other departmental employees. The department directors are present during the initial meeting and they can reinforce the importance of the project to other department members.

In addition to the survey form, departmental team members are responsible for completing 10 data dictionary contents forms (see Table 5G). They will complete one form for each of the 10 MPI data elements in their systems. If their systems do not have one of the data elements (eg, occupation), they are to return the form with the statement "Not in department system."

Give the team members two weeks to complete their forms. In the interim, it is likely that they will need clarification on some of the data elements and their formats and rules. Questions should be addressed to the project leader, who can get further assistance from the database administrator. Occasionally, the answers to some of the questions can be obtained from the departmental system documentation or directly from the vendor.

The team members should bring their completed forms to the second meeting. The forms are reviewed and compared with the ASTM standards and the team members discuss the relationships of their data to the core data during the next two weeks. At the third meeting, the group will review the final results of the departmental forms and their relationships to the core data dictionary file.

Database system requirements and selection
Concurrent with the departmental data collection process, the next step for the

TABLE 5H - Data Dictionary Database Application Specifications		
Quality	**Definition**	**Criteria Met**
Portable	Device independent, able to transfer from one technological environment to another	
Reliable	System has protections from internal and external disruption	
Flexible	Has general applicability and can be modified	
Efficient	Optimal use of computer time and storage	
User friendly	Easy for users to input, view, and query	
Maintainable	Simple to design and change	
Robust	Meets current and near-future needs	
Adaptable	Presents varying user views and queries	

project leader and database administrator is to design and select the database software on which to store the data dictionary.

There are four crucial points to remember in designing the data dictionary database:
- It needs to be relatively easy to use and to teach to others.

- The entry of the data must be easy and quick and encourage accuracy.
- Reports should be uncomplicated, yet accommodate user's requests.
- The database must be flexible and easy to modify.

Make the data dictionary database as simple as possible; pattern each departmental table after the survey forms. Design a data dictionary that provides for easy entry and updating; it must be useful to those who are making queries of it. A vital component of any well designed database is that it be flexible; in the health care environment, this means that it must be able to accommodate such changes as the addition of a new laboratory system, a computerized data set for long-term care reporting, or an entire new billing system. You want it to remain useful and manageable in the years to come as you continue to build a CPR or participate in a CHIN.

Use databases that comply with industry standards such as Xbase or SQL and choose database software that can move to another hardware platform. The database should work on a stand-alone PC, in a distributed processing environment (client server), or on the mainframe. If you eventually plan to move the data dictionary from a passive to an active type (see Chapter 1), it must be capable of connecting with the separate databases of the organization. Table 5H lists some of the key qualities that a user-friendly database should have, and Sidebar 5A discusses your software options.

At this point in the project you should have decided which computer systems and data elements your project will include, how much time and money it will take, how the database will be designed, and what software package you will use. Now you are ready to implement the data dictionary.

SIDEBAR 5A - Selecting Database Software

Selection of the database software for the data dictionary is very much an organizational decision. You may pick a system with which your database administrator is already familiar, or a system that you've already licensed for use elsewhere in the facility. You can choose either a desktop system or an enterprise-wide system.

Desktop systems are PC-based. Microsoft Access, Borland's Paradox, and a PC-based version of Oracle are all examples of popular desktop database systems. The advantages of this type of system include portability (so any department can easily install and use a similar system), frequent product updates, and plenty of people who know the software.

Enterprise-wide systems are usually Unix based and allow for more users. They have more complex, network-based software that prevents concurrent users from interfering with each other. These systems include Oracle, Sybase, Watcom, Informix, and Microsoft's SQL server.

The database for our data dictionary project is written in Microsoft Access. We chose Access because it allows a visual look at the data and offers simple ways to view and work with the information that is generated. It has good query tools, and can connect data regardless of the format or location. Queries can be changed and different layouts are easy to see. Access uses WYSIWYG (what you see is what you get) design tools to produce forms and reports in a readable format. It also has "wizards," which walk a novice user through steps and macros and a database programming language for more technical users.

Chapter 6

Implementing the Data Dictionary

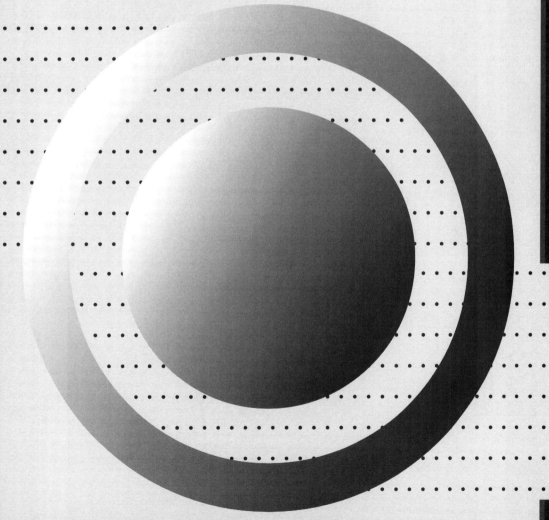

Chapter 6
Implementing the Data Dictionary

After the project team members from each department have surveyed their departmental systems and returned with the selected data elements and their associated attributes, the implementation of this type of data dictionary is a very simple process. Since it is a passive data dictionary and not an active type (see description in Chapter 1 for a reminder of the difference) the data dictionary implementation is not dependent on data from any other system nor does it update data in other systems. The processes involved in the implementation include:

- designing the database tables, forms, and reports,
- addressing any issues that have surfaced,
- training the users,
- conducting a project review, and
- documenting the project in a final report.

General database design principles

We have worked through a project example in Chapter 5. Below are some general database design principles. For most organizations the initial database will be quite simple, with a small number of data tables. Looking at the example from Chapter 5, most, if not all, of the data tables will have the same exact structure.

Table design

A database administrator can make this part of your project much easier. In general, table structure should be designed using standard database rules that are found in texts on database design. There are two important rules to remember when designing the tables.

1. *The entity integrity rule—each row in each table must always have a primary-key value.*

For this project, this means that in each of the departmental tables, the first column (or attribute) for each data element is the ASTM number. This is why the ASTM numbers were chosen, because each number uniquely identifies an individual data element.

2. *The primary-key integrity rule—a primary key must be unique within a table, ie, not repeated in any other row.*

This rule is easy to obey—just list the ASTM number once. This rule comes into play in more complicated databases but it doesn't hurt to mention it here.

Forms

A form is a "user view"—a simple, visual representation of data elements that allows the user to perform a specific function, such as data entry, without any knowledge of the underlying maze of tables, primary keys, and the like. The database administrator will need to develop screen forms for data entry and data update, especially if tables are maintained and updated by nontechnical or clerical people. Forms force the data entry process to conform to edit rules that have been established. For instance, in Figure 6A, the field PATIENT NAME is shown. For the attribute "Length," the database administrator has coded this as a numeric field so when a user enters a value in this field, it must be a number or it will not be accepted. Having forms with edit rules such as this helps to keep inconsistent data out of the database.

For the last three fields, "Responsibility," "Update Authority," and "Final Authority," the database administrator has added a "drop down box" that accesses the contents of a small table called "Department Name" (see Table 6A). This table identifies different departments and assigns them a three-character code; eg, REG is the registration department. This feature contributes to the consistency of data entered into the tables by forcing users to use a department naming scheme.

This project is structured to allow the departmental users to enter data into the data dictionary database themselves. The rationale for this is that if the users

FIGURE 6A - ADT Table Input Form

ASTM Number:	01001
Field Name:	PATIENT_NAME
Field Code:	Patients Name
Description:	Person receiving health care services and about whom records containing data about those services are collected
Synonyms:	NA
Source:	AST, NURS
Format Type:	text
Lexicon Used:	N/A
Length:	30
Allowable Range:	N/A
Confidentiality Level:	2
Access Level:	2
Edits:	Last name comma space first name
Responsibility:	REG
Update Authority:	NUR
Final Authority:	HIM

TABLE 6A - Department Name

ID	Department	Department Name
1	NUR	Nursing
2	HIM	Health Information Management
3	REG	Registration
4	PHA	Pharmacy
5	RAD	Radiology
6	LAB	Laboratory
7	PAA	Patient Accounts
8	DSS	Decision Support
9	CMX	Case Mix
10	TUR	Tumor Registry
11	BIR	Birth Registry
12	TRA	Trauma Registry
13	DET	Dietary
14	PTT	Physical Medicine
15	OTT	Occupational Medicine
16	OPR	Operating Room
17	ASC	Ambulatory Surgery Center
18	MNH	Mental Health
19	MIS	Medical Information System
20	PTH	Pathology

are responsible for maintaining their own system data table, they will stay involved and interested in further development of the data dictionary. This approach makes sense when:

- there are a limited number of data elements to enter;
- the database is designed to be simple enough for any computer user to enter data; and
- the database is accessible on the network or users can easily access the database on a centralized computer.

Reports

The database administrator should develop standard reports. At least one report will be used to audit the table data entry done by the users. As shown in Figure 6B, this report allows the database administrator to quickly scan the data entry done by the pharmacy system. This report shows that the "Description" appears to have been entered incorrectly. The database administrator can routinely run this report and give the output to the project leader who can then have the pharmacy team member complete the data entry.

Other reports are designed to meet information needs of team members, other users, and organization management. Get input from the team and end users about what information is important to them and how they would like to see it presented. For example, the patient billing department may be interested in a report that lists all computer systems having the PATIENT NAME field, whether it is called NAME, SUBSCRIBER NAME, FULL NAME, or CUSTOMER NAME. This would help clarify problems with names that are transferred from other computer systems in a different format than is acceptable to the patient billing system (see Figure 6C).

You will not design many reports during the implementation phase. As the data dictionary grows and as the organization learns what the data dictionary is for, there will be new requests. Microsoft Access has report wizards to walk novice users through the steps of designing new reports. Remember, the reason you put data into a database is so it can be retrieved and used. Promote your data dictionary by accommodating your users' requests; the more you use this database, the more it will be used by others.

Implementation issues

The passive data dictionary is designed in a simple database format, so there are very few things that can go wrong with the software during implementation. Anything that does go wrong with the software is easily remedied by the database administrator, who understands database design and operation. Because there are no interfaces with other computer systems, there is a low degree of risk if this database does not operate properly to start with; there is a very high

FIGURE 6B - Audit Report

PHARMACY DATA DICTIONARY CONTENTS

Field Name Description	ASTM Num	Field Code	Synonyms	Data Type	Length	Date added	Initials
DOB	01032	PersBirthDtm	DOB Date of Birth	date	8	1/1/97	**MRH**
The exact time of the birth							
FAMILY_MEMBER_FEMALE_PARENT_MAIDEN_NAME	01090.11	FAMMbrFemaleParentName	Mother's Maiden Name	text	33	1/1/97	**MRH**
The name of the biologic....							
HOME_PHONE	01100	PersHomePhoneNum	Telephone Number	numeric	10	1/1/97	**MRH**
The phone num...							
OCCUPATION	01065	OccOccupationName	Patient Occupation	numeric	14	1/1/97	**MRH**
The employment, business, or a course of action in which the patient is engaged (i.e., student)							

FIGURE 6C - User Request Report

DATA DICTIONARY DATABASE REPORT

Generated For: Patient Billing

Data Generated: 1-1-97

Request: List all departments containing ASTM #01001 (Patient Name) and all synonyms

DEPARTMENT NAME	SYNONYMS FOR PATIENT NAME
Decision Support	N/A
Health Information	Patient's full name
Nursing	N/A
Laboratory	Full name
Pharmacy	Customer name
Radiology	N/A
Registration	Full name, legal name, patient's full name, subscriber name
Patient billing	Legal name

probability that any problems can be quickly resolved. That's the good news about a project of this type.

The bad news is that there are all kinds of other problems that can occur throughout the project that might cause it to stall or, worse yet, to stop altogether. Throughout the book you have been encouraged to plan so that you can avoid some of the major problems.

- If the administration is not committed to this project and its ongoing maintenance, the project may get delayed in favor of other initiatives that they do support. Keep up your communication by informing the administrative sponsor of progress along the way.

- There are practically tens of thousands of data elements that you can define. Many organizations bite off more than they can chew and become overwhelmed. The bigger the project, the less likely it is to be finished. Discipline yourself to limit the initial number of data elements. Don't get ahead of yourself when adding additional data elements.

- Labor dollars are decreasing as health care goes through a seemingly never ending belt tightening process. Use your project time wisely by setting up a firm foundation on which the data dictionary can grow. Once the organization understands that a data dictionary is an important part of information management, adding new data elements will become part of the day-to-day activities.

Additional problems can be loosely categorized into communication, sponsorship, scope, priorities, and system. Table 6B outlines these general types of problems and some adaptive actions you can take.

Training

Training is the key to the ongoing success of the project. Good training helps keep members involved and contributing. Since a data dictionary is never

TABLE 6B - Common Problems and Solutions		
Problem Type Potential Issue	**Problem Description**	**Adaptive Action Suggested Solution or Approach**
COMMUNICATION	Lack of awareness	Increase communication
	Complacency	Provide further education about problems and benefits
	Non-performers	Use regular feedback, meetings, one-on-one communication
SPONSORSHIP	Organizational barriers	Enlist administrative sponsor assistance
	Lack of upper management support	Include sponsor in kick-off, update administration with communications about milestones and successes
	Management may not be committed to the data dictionary project and its ongoing maintenance	Clearly establish and define the project objective and its tie-in with the IM plan
	Too little authority for project leader	Define roles and responsibilities
	Empire building/ protection	Involve or communicate regularly with department managers

Problem Type Potential Issue	Problem Description	Adaptive Action Suggested Solution or Approach
SPONSORSHIP (continued)	Lack of commitment	Provide project plan/overview to reinforce importance Match project objectives with sponsor's personal needs
	Poor team member involvement	Perform team building exercises Clarify roles and responsibilities Train and develop team members
SCOPE	Inadequate planning	Develop plan that includes acknowledgment of other current organizational projects (accreditation surveys, mergers, reorganizations, administrative turnover) Establish project schedule and budget Define project scope

TABLE 6B - Common Problems and Solutions (continued)

TABLE 6B - Common Problems and Solutions (continued)		
Problem Type Potential Issue	**Problem Description**	**Adaptive Action Suggested Solution or Approach**
SCOPE (continued)	Inadequate planning (continued)	Solicit departmental and user needs through departmental surveys Determine staffing requirements
PRIORITIES (TIME)	Impact on productivity	Limit scope
	Unexpected conflicts for time	Reinforce that investment of time in project now will yield organizational benefits and save time and money in the long run Clearly define objective and use administrative sponsor to reinforce project priority
	Inability to estimate target dates	Use project plan to outline time frames Incorporate departments' data needs into project to get departmental buy-in and interest in project completion

TABLE 6B - Common Problems and Solutions (continued)

Problem Type Potential Issue	Problem Description	Adaptive Action Suggested Solution or Approach
PRIORITIES (continued)	Inability to estimate target dates (continued)	Track progress and update schedules
		Acknowledge milestones reached
		Establish contingency plans
SYSTEM	Data coming from the departmental systems is inaccurate	Run audit report frequently and provide further training or assistance to team member having problems
	Lack of information about a departmental system	Contact system vendor
	Poor database selection	Use new database because of low cost of desktop systems

complete, in order for it to be a vital part of the organization, it must be constantly changing. This is further discussed in Chapter 7; in short, new data elements will be added, new departmental systems will be included, and new computer systems will be integrated into the organization. The data dictionary will remain viable if users access and use the data dictionary system; to ensure that this happens, users must be well trained.

First and foremost, users must understand the project, its impact on the organization, and their contribution to the project's success. When people are well trained and understand what they are doing, they are more likely to maintain the data dictionary. This overall understanding is virtually guaranteed by using the team approach to the data dictionary project. As team members participate in the unfolding of the project, they gain understanding, an essential objective of good training. This ensures that the users are invested in the data dictionary and will be strong champions for its use in the organization.

Users must learn to perform the basic mechanics of data entry and simple report generation. Outline a training program that covers what people need to learn, how they will be taught, how their performance will be evaluated, when they will be trained, and who will train them. The project leader and database administrator should train the users. A training program for the departmental team members should occur during weeks 9 and 10 of the project and include the following:

- Content
    - Collect departmental data
    - Enter data into database
    - Generate canned reports
    - Generate simple ad hoc reports

- Methodology
    - Train classes of users in computer learning center
    - Utilize test system

- Performance goals
    - Independently collect departmental system data for new data elements
    - Enter data into database with no errors
    - Generate reports with no assistance

Managers are trained to query the database, use canned reports, and create simple ad hoc reports. Managers are best trained in one-on-one sessions to avoid possible fear of failure in front of their peers. Remember, these people need to see the value of this project so that they will ensure their department users maintain the data dictionary.

It is important that the users have some practice time with the system before they start to use it on the job. This is best done just before they will enter real data or request reports that they need. If training is done too early, users will most likely forget exactly what to do and they may become discouraged. After the project ends, ongoing training may or may not be necessary. Periodically solicit feedback from the members who participated on the team and other users to determine if there is a need for additional training. Also, if the audit reports show an increasing error rate, this is a clear signal that some follow-up training is needed.

Document your training efforts to show that your organization is complying with the JCAHO IM.4 Standard, which states "Decision makers and other individuals in the organization who generate, collect, analyze and use information are educated and trained in information management principles." The training done for the data dictionary project is an excellent opportunity to demonstrate that the producers and users of information are improving the quality of the organization's information resources.

Project review and wrap-up

At the end of the project, it is good business practice to document your work in a final report. The project review done in the wrap-up meeting will provide much of the material for the report. Prepare a summary of activities of the project using the process lists and any progress reports you have prepared. If the review points out problems, the database administrator can still make the necessary changes because you've created a simple database. Your review will assist in answering questions from administration such as, "Were the project objectives achieved?", "Is the data dictionary what you had envisioned?", and "Are there any undesirable effects?".

The objective of the project in this book is to implement a data dictionary for a core set of data elements and eight designated departments using ASTM standards. The implementation serves to comply with the JCAHO IM 3 Standard and to begin to better standardize data in preparation for the implementation of a CPR. The project was to have been completed within a 12-week period and was not to exceed a budget of $18,450.

Using the final report format in Table 6C, document the project and its product, the data dictionary. Reiterate the project objective and briefly describe the resulting data dictionary. An honest project review will point out the areas that need corrective action and will give advice about future efforts.

Congratulations! You have completed your project. At this point the team disbands and the project becomes a daily activity, owned by the respective departments and the information systems department. The data dictionary is a powerful tool that can help your organization move from data disorganization to information management, but you must keep it going. Although the formal data dictionary project is over, you can be instrumental in planning for additions, changes, and deletions in the database. Chapter 7 will help you prepare for ongoing development.

TABLE 6C - Final Report—Data Dictionary Project

_____(Project Leader Name)
_____(Report Date)
_____(Time period covered)

TEAM MEMBERS

EXECUTIVE SUMMARY/OVERVIEW

Brief paragraph or 5–7 bullet points
Project objective
Data dictionary description

ACCOMPLISHMENTS

Milestones reached
Changes in project

PROJECT ANALYSIS

Problems and corrective actions
Changes to project and rationale
Unresolved issues and proposed resolutions

TABLE 6C - Final Report—Data Dictionary Project (continued)

ONGOING MAINTENANCE AND BUILDING

Future considerations
New data elements
New departments
Changed data elements
New computer systems

_____
_____
_____

RECOMMENDATIONS

Advice about future efforts

_____
_____
_____

ATTACHMENTS

Screen shots, tables, reports

Chapter 6

Notes

Chapter 7
Ongoing Development

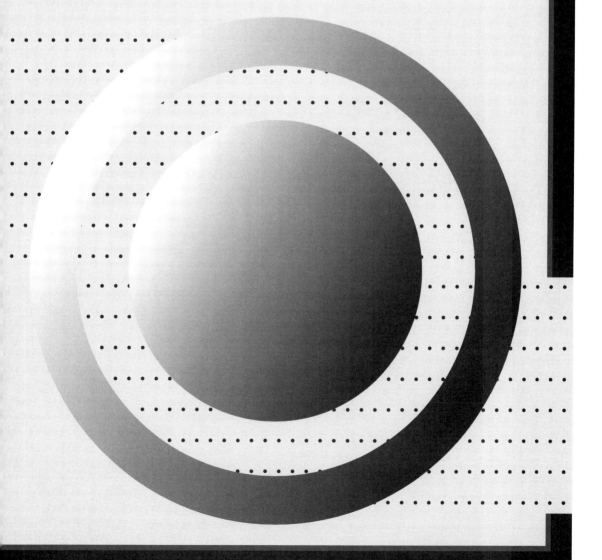

Chapter 7
Ongoing Development

This book discusses the importance of using a data dictionary to ensure the production of accurate data. This in turn is used to generate quality information, which gives a health care organization the competitive business advantage necessary to survive in a rapidly growing information age. The project in Chapters 5 and 6 shows how a health care organization can define the scope of a data dictionary, delineate tasks and responsibilities, and plan, design, and implement the initial data elements for a data dictionary. The next step, discussed here in Chapter 7, is to build on the success of the project by adding new data elements for the project departments, by adding new departments, and by insisting on the use of standard data definitions when new computer systems are added.

Therefore, the completed project in Chapters 5 and 6 becomes a model upon which the organization continues to build its dynamic data dictionary. This project data set contains 10 important data elements that are used to uniquely identify patients and are routinely contained in most clinical computer systems. How does an organization decide which data elements to add next?

Priority levels for ongoing development

Figure 7A shows a logical approach an organization can take in deciding which data elements are critical and should be standardized next. There are four levels of prioritization. The first level of priority is to standardize data elements that are regulated. The second level includes data elements that are part of widely accepted standards. The third contains data found in the facility's computer systems and the fourth level, the most difficult, is to try to predict what is needed for the future. Each priority level is discussed below.

Level one: *Required standards*
The first level of priority includes some of the health care industry regulatory

Chapter 7

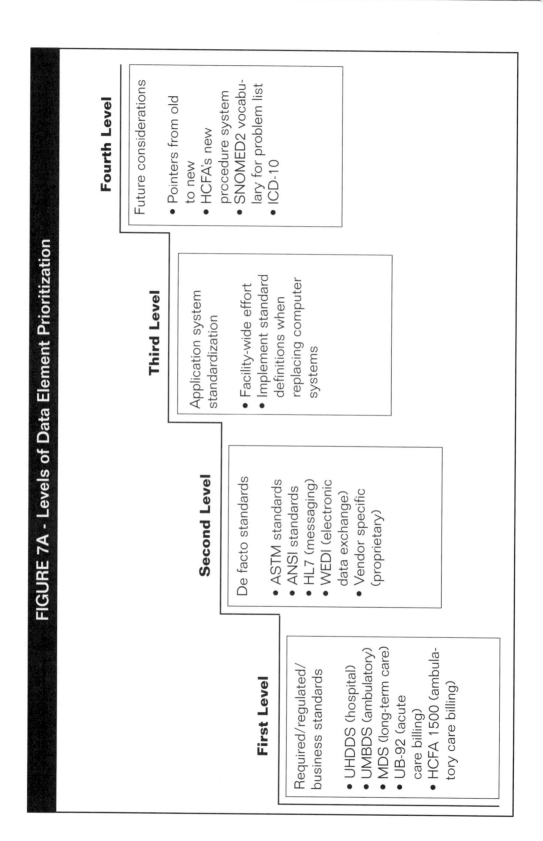

standards and delineates required or regulated data elements. These data definitions are used in various types of data transfer and must be adhered to when submitting data. A facility has no choice but to comply with these data definitions when they are sending out data in reports or on billing forms. Because the definitions for these data elements are mandatory, it makes sense to add these to the data dictionary.

For example, clinics use the HCFA-1500 Health Insurance Claim Form to bill Medicare and many other insurers. Two data elements on this form are "Date of Current Illness MM DD YY, (first symptom) or Injury, or Pregnancy (last menstrual period)" and "If Patient Has Had Same or Similar Illness Give First Date MM DD YY." A clinic should add these data elements to its data dictionary.

Level two: de facto standards

The second level illustrates some de facto standards, or those standards that are accepted by the health care industry. The standards organizations, referred to in the introduction, are developing technical, procedural, and systems standards and guidelines and industry practices necessary to support the development of the CPR. For example, the Health Record Core Data Set was developed by the American Health Information Management (AHIMA) Council on Professional Practice to create a core data set as the foundation of an integrated clinical and financial patient information system (see Table 7A).

Many large vendors have built data dictionaries into their computer systems. Although these definitions relate only to their proprietary systems, they are widely used and therefore can provide a stepping-stone in building the facility's own data dictionary.

Level three: Application system standardization

The third level, that of defining data elements throughout all computer systems in the organization, should be approached only after building a firm foundation of data definitions—otherwise the project will be overwhelming. Once you have a set of data definitions, and a plan for adding to the data dictionary, progress by adding one data definition at a time. Work "ahead of

TABLE 7A - Health Record Core Data Set

1. Patient's number (personal identification)
2. Patient's name
3. Date of birth
4. Address/Residence
5. Sex
6. Race
7. Social Security Number
8. Patient's home phone number
9. Patient's work phone number
10. Marital status
11. Name of legal next of kin
12. Address of next of kin
13. Name of guarantor
14. Address of guarantor
15. Religion
16. Occupation
17. Employer name
18. Employer address
19. Principal source of payment
20. Insurance group number
21. Attending provider (physician) name
22. Date of encounter/admission (commencement of service, service date)
23. Hour of admission
24. Place of encounter
25. Admission source
26. Hospital/Provider identification number
27. Admission type
28. Operating physician
29. Reason for encounter
30. Allergies
31. Diagnostic services
32. Therapeutic services
33. Admission diagnosis
34. Principal diagnosis
35. Additional (other, secondary) diagnoses
36. Discharge date
37. Discharge hour
38. Disposition
39. Principal procedure
40. Principal procedure date
41. Other procedure code(s)
42. Other procedure date
43. Total length of stay
44. Total charges
45. Total costs

From Journal of AHIMA, December 1986, page 48

time" and insist that new computer applications use standardized data definitions to make additions to the data dictionary an easier task. This is discussed more at the end of this chapter.

Level four: Future considerations
A fourth level is added to alert the data dictionary project leader to stay current in health care trends and new computing innovations. The project leader must try to forecast the future. What will happen to old ICD-9-CM procedure codes when HCFA implements its new procedure system? How will you map ICD-9-CM codes to ICD-10 codes? What if SNOMED 2 is used as vocabulary for the clinic's problem lists? How will a facility map the old DRG system to a severity-adjusted DRG system? These questions cannot be answered now but must be considered in the future, especially when planning for additions to the data dictionary.

Building the data dictionary
Ongoing data dictionary development must focus on at least three areas. The participants in the initial project will be adding new data elements and will occasionally need to change a data element's definition. Some of these departments have more than one computer system and they need to create new tables for these systems and to relate them to the core table. New departments should contribute to the building of the data dictionary to keep the database alive and well. Lastly, as new computer systems are incorporated into the organization, the data elements need to be reconciled with or added to the data dictionary.

Adding departmental data elements
The departments that were involved initially in the design, building, and implementation of the facility's data dictionary are the likely candidates to continue its development. They have learned why a data dictionary is important, have helped design one, and have been trained on the data entry requirements and reporting capabilities. They will now look at their own data elements and computer interfaces and understand more about data exchange. They will know where to begin their investigation when problems occur with data moving into and out of their computer system.

New data elements

Referring to Figure 7A, your organization may outline a plan to define all the regulated data elements in the first priority level. In some states, the registration department is required to enter the race of a patient who is being admitted to the hospital. The clinic at a teaching facility would also benefit by adding "race" to their data set if they are doing population studies. To add the data element RACE to the ADT data dictionary table, the registration department representative first contacts the data dictionary database administrator requesting that this data element be added. The registration department representative then receives the ASTM number, the field name, field code, and ASTM description:

> 01042 RACE PersRaceCode "The major biologic class to which the patient belongs as a result of a pedigree analysis or with which the patient identifies him/her self in cases where the data are not conclusive."

The database administrator adds this data element to the core table and the department representative gathers the attributes of the data element using a form similar to that shown in Table 5G. He or she subsequently enters the ASTM number and data element attributes into the registration data dictionary table.

To ensure ongoing additions and growth of the data dictionary, set up a committee structure whereby participating departments meet regularly to decide which data elements they all need to define. The committee structure is similar to a Forms Committee, and if the data elements being added are clinical, these data elements would be a regular item for discussion by the Medical Record Committee.

Other systems within a department

Some departments have more than one computer system. An example is the Health Information Management department, where the following computer systems are common:

- Master Patient Index
- Coding and abstracting
- Chart deficiency, location, and tracking
- Birth certificate registry
- Dictation
- Transcription
- Trauma registry
- Oncology cancer registry

An organization may decide that they want to have each of the participating departments further define the core data elements in every one of their departmental computer systems. The process for doing this would be the same as the initial process of using the ASTM core definitions and creating a new table for each computer system as discussed in Chapter 5.

Changed data elements
Occasionally a data element's definition will change. Although this will be a rare occurrence, you should define a process for changing the definition. The department representative would talk with the database administrator in advance of the change. The database administrator can assess the impact of the change on the whole data dictionary and on other departments and computer systems. The department representative would define the changed attributes, again using a form similar to Table 5G, and enter these into the database.

The database administrator keeps the original definition for historical reference and as an audit trail. The change is communicated to all participating departments through a memorandum, e-mail, or report generated from the data dictionary database.

Adding new departments
Referring again to Table 7A, add departments based on who contributes any data to the required standards. If you are part of a health care system and have a long-term–care facility, add a representative from this area who will con-

tribute new data elements to the data dictionary. Once you have finished with the first level, look at the second level and continue to add more data elements. Depending on your organization's size this can keep you busy for years, but again, this is an ongoing process.

An alternative approach to adding new departments is to choose to add departments that interface with, or transmit data to and from, those departments that were involved in the initial project. As a matter of fact, the participating departments will have strong opinions about which departments should be next, based on problems they are having with data transmission. These data problems will point to new department participants for the data dictionary.

Physical medicine may be registering patients for ongoing therapy; patient billing has complained that these registrars chronically omit the date of injury during their initial registration process. Since this data element is required for the bill, the patient account reps must request the information from the referring physician's office. Adding the physical medicine department to the data dictionary process begins the communication process, which leads to data standardization and data integrity.

Adding new computer systems

When a health care organization is choosing and installing a new computer system, there is a unique opportunity to work with vendors. Legacy systems, or systems that have been around for years, are difficult, if not impossible, to change. The best you can hope for is to "point" the data elements to the core data definitions and hope that any new interfaces go well. When you swap out these legacy systems, as is discussed in the case study in Chapter 8, you can ensure that data from the proposed system is defined in the same manner as the core data definitions. Sure it takes work, but if there is hope for true application system standardization it is at this point.

RFPs and contracts
Include the data definitions in your Request For Proposal (RFP) when you are seeking new systems. Since you have started with a core set of data elements

that are important to the facility, you can instruct the vendor on how to design the data structures. Also include language in the RFP or contract that requires the vendor to continue to work with you as new data elements are defined. This is a great opportunity to see how flexible a vendor's software really is. If they tell you they can't easily make these changes, take a better look at other, more adaptable vendors.

Working with installation teams
Working with the installation teams will be a challenge. Many times, the sales process promises anything you ask for, but when the real work begins, the installation people may tell you it is too hard to change their software program coding. Pull out the RFP and contract and remind them of their promises. You can always compromise if you need to, by accepting their design and matching it with the core table, but don't tell them that until they have tried to adapt their definitions. Remember, the goal is the management of information resources through standardization of data. Don't back down too easily.

Planning for future needs

The health care industry is in the midst of tremendous change and in order to remain competitive, an organization must be able to plan for the future. The computer systems must be well designed, flexible, and able to accommodate the rapid changes. Whether your organization is planning to computerize a single departmental function, to implement a fully functional CPR, or to participate in a CHIN, you must develop a strategic plan that will support the information needs of the future.

Strategic thinking about information resources includes working with organizational goals and translating these into specific goals and objectives for the management of data and information. Chapter 8 is a case study on an organization that has done just that. They have decided as an organization that data is an important asset—just as important as financial viability. They have determined the resources they require, established policies and procedures for the use of these resources, and woven a data dictionary into the fabric of their data management plan.

Notes

Chapter 8
Case Study

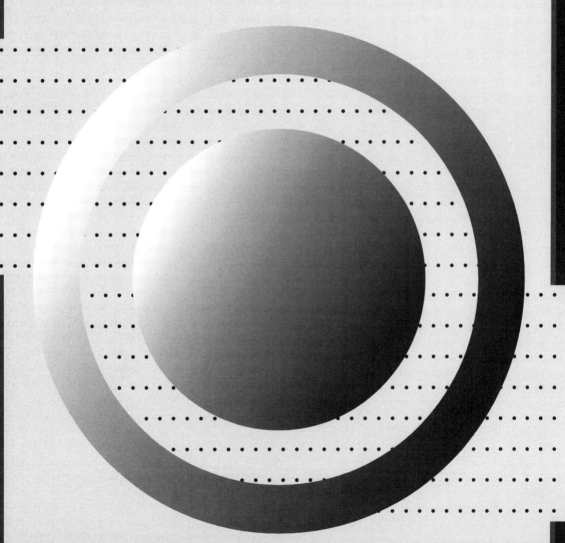

Chapter 8
Case Study

This case study describes how Holy Cross Health System Corporation (HCHSC) uses a data dictionary as part of their overall strategic business plan. HCHSC operates in six distinct markets throughout the United States. Its seven member organizations include acute-care hospitals, extended care facilities, residential centers for the disabled and elderly, ambulatory care and surgery centers, clinics for the poor, community service organizations, an ambulatory management company, a college of nursing, home health and hospice programs, and preferred provider organizations. The size of the HCHSC system requires a different approach to data dictionary development and management than the 12-week project we describe in this book, but the same principles apply to smaller and single-focus facilities.

The seven member organizations vary in size and scope. They are located in different geographical areas, serve six different markets, and grapple with different state regulations. Each member has its own database, but all the member databases reside in HCHSC' main location for easier management. Together, these databases, along with external data, comprise a "decision support system" for HCHSC. The system contains nine years of archived historical data and six years of current online data. It all adds up to a large, complex system serving the various needs of multiple customers. The decision support system contains a data dictionary running under ADABAS software (produced by Software AG.).

When to Build a Data Dictionary

HCHSC initially began their data dictionary project during the process of changing their legacy financial systems and choosing new software for patient accounting and accounts receivable. These two financial applications provide a large share of the data to the decision support system. But before their corporate Information Resources department could build a data dictionary, they had to answer the following questions:

- What are the most important areas of information to address?
- How can we best meet the information needs of a diverse health care system?
- How can we properly manage data to ensure that our information is accurate, reliable, valid, and complete?
- How can we make this information available to the right people at the right time?

The Key to Success

As we discussed in Chapter 3, successful data dictionary projects depend on the support of upper management. At HCHSC, upper management considers accurate, integrated data as critical to the organization's success. With this charge, their Information Resources department promotes data standardization with the members as a way of life, not as a one-time project owned by a project manager. This philosophy makes it easier to convince the whole organization to buy into the importance of data standards.

Planning and designing

Information Resources first wrote policies and procedures that addressed the management of data as a strategic asset. These policies and procedures also addressed the standardization of data. To identify important data elements, they created a matrix that established the information requirements for an integrated delivery system (IDS).

In designing the matrix, HCHSC looked at it from the member organizations' standpoint, as each member organization needs data and information to manage business in its own local market. Information Resources worked with the Chief Information Officers from each organization to fulfill their specific data and information needs.

Information Resources concentrated on functional areas with high information needs, such as finance, human resources, corporate development, strategic planning, managed care, and contracting. They asked people to look at the data from a historical perspective, analyze the current requirements and forecast future needs. The goals were to pick out which data elements were most important to the member organizations and to the corporation, and determine what value-added processes were necessary to create other critical data (ie, cost accounting).

These data and information needs were then ranked as

- mission critical,
- important, or
- nice to have.

The mission critical needs were addressed first. Some of the mission critical needs include:

- Addition of data elements as industry requirements change and grow
- Software programs to generate new reports
- Online capabilities so users can query and use the decision support database
- Addition of external database with risk adjustments/severity scoring

Because payers and the government are the biggest outside recipients of data, HCHSC also included standards from the UB-92 and HCFA 1500 billing sets; these data elements became de facto standards (see Chapter 7) with which they began to build their data definitions. They could then choose other data elements that were important to their own business needs.

Although they used national standards such as ASTM and HL7 to define their data elements, they used each member's system requirements to define attributes (such as field length and format type). In other words, one member's computer system defines race using a field length of two numeric characters and another system uses three alpha-numeric characters; field length varies according to the vendor's system formatting. Information Resources then linked the various definitions between the systems, similar to the example in this book of the core data definitions linked through the ASTM number to the data elements in the departmental computer systems.

Components of the Data Dictionary

There are more than 2,000 data items defined in the HCHSC decision support system. Of these, there are over 600 data elements, or objects, defined for the user (or customer) to access in HCHSC' decision support system. Over one hundred of these elements also are identified as critical and are defined as "Patient Financial Systems Data Standards." These include data elements such as:

- Patient name
- Patient birth date
- Patient address
- Patient gender
- Patient insurance
- Patient employer
- Referring physician
- Diagnoses (up to 15 occurrences)
- Dates of services
- Patient account number

There are many other important data elements in the decision support system that have not yet been included in the data standards development, but are still available for creating reports across the health care system. These elements include patient identifying data such as medical record number, social security number, and Medicare number.

Data Standards Analyst

Just as upper management support is key to get a data dictionary project started, a data standards analyst is key to keep it going. This person must thoroughly understand the data and data relationships of each member's system and incorporate established data standards into each new computer system as it comes online. The analyst meets with representatives in the member organizations to define the data elements they feel are beneficial to their organization and to the corporation as a whole. This also includes working with vendors to ensure that they design and install new systems according to the data standardization policies.

The data standards analyst also can provide additional information to help the member organizations, such as the name of the data element in the data dictionary, where it is physically located within the file (ie, what file segment), the source of the element, and whether the data element is user entered, interfaced, or derived. Those who use the data and information often need to go to the source of the data to rectify discrepancies or to discuss the addition of new data elements.

Reports

At the corporate level, system and management reports are run to keep track of data. Audit reports are designed to verify that data is flowing correctly through the interfaces, or to look at total dollars and total counts. The member organizations can get to the data by running queries; they can design and generate their own reports using the data to show profitability, gather market information, or track trends. Information Resources assists with more complicated reports and also provides assistance with expert statistical analysis.

Ongoing development

HCHSC feels that an ideal time to implement data standards is during the swapping out of legacy systems. They insist on implementing the data management policies as systems are acquired and not later through "retrofitting". This work begins when they write the RFP (request for proposal) which specifies that the data standards will be used during implementation. Language concerning data standards is also included in the contract and in the model implementation plan. This constantly reinforces the importance of standards.

The commitment they had obtained earlier from their member organizations was crucial to making data standardization successful. They have found that it requires continued dedication to keep it going, but they find it rewarding to see the effectiveness of a data dictionary defined with standards. The organization is clearly reaping benefits from this ongoing project.

Resources & Glossary of Database Management Terms

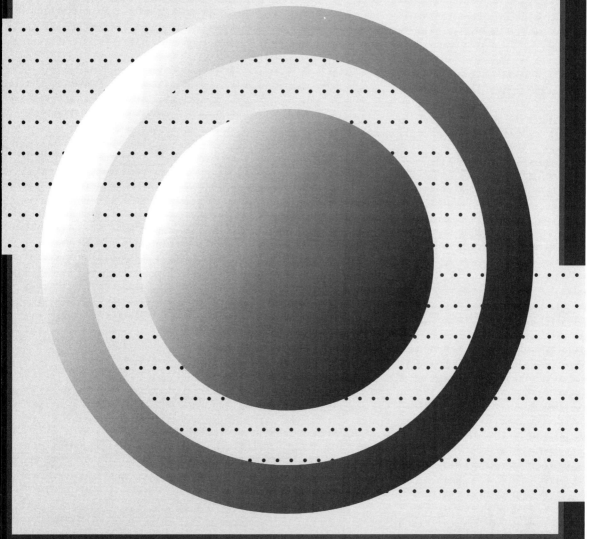

Resources

Effective meetings

Covey, Stephen R., *The Seven Habits of Highly Effective People*, Simon and Schuster, New York NY, 1989

Doyle, Michael and Straus, David, *How to Make Meetings Work: the New Interactive Method*, Wyden Books, New York NY, 1976

Lewis, James P., *Project Planning, Scheduling and Control*, Probus Publishing Co., Chicago IL, 1991

Marshall, Lisa and Friedman, Lucy, *Smart Work: The Syntax Guide for Mutual Understanding in the Workplace*, Kendall/Hunt Publishing Co., Dubuque IA, 1995

Standards

ASTM (American Society for Testing and Materials) E 1384 - 96 Standard Guide for Content and Structure of the Computer-Based Patient Record April 1996, [order from] ASTM, 100 Barr Harbor Dr., West Conshohocken, PA 19428

CPR

Dick, Richard S. and Steen, Elaine B., *The Computer-based Patient Record: An Essential Technology for Health Care*, National Academy Press, Washington DC, 1991

Health Information Management

Huffman, Edna K. *Health Information Management*, Physicians' Record Company, Berwyn IL, 1994

Notes

A Glossary of Database Management Terms

Application program
A computer program that performs one task or set of tasks, associated with one particular application.

Application system
An integrated group of application programs, procedures, and data files that perform processes or functions.

Data
Discrete facts about people, places, things, events, or concepts recorded on paper or on magnetic or optical media.

Data aggregate
A collection of data items that are named and referenced as a whole; eg, NAME includes LAST NAME, FIRST NAME, and MIDDLE INITIAL. When data aggregates are used, they must also be defined in the DD. Their entry in the DD would list data aggregate name, description, and names of included data items.

Database
An integrated, interrelated collection of data for use in generating shared information. A database stores information that is important to an organization and allows concurrent access by multiple users for a variety of purposes.
A well organized database reduces redundancy, increases consistency, and reduces wasted storage space. There is therefore less time spent investigating and unraveling errors and reporting variability.

Database administrator (DBA)
The person responsible for defining an organization's data resources.

Responsibilities include working with users to define their own data, modeling the data, designing databases, developing edits and controls, and evaluating new database software products and emerging technologies for handling information.

Database management system (DBMS)
A general software system that manages requests for data. It provides access to data for multiple users and maintains an audit trail or log of all activities.

Data communication
The exchange of digital forms of data or information between two locations or systems.

Data definition
A statement conveying the fundamental nature of a data element including use, size, type, content, format, access, ownership, source, and additional facts. Data definition allows organizations to more effectively manage their information resources.

Data definition (or description) language (DDL)
The lexicon used by a database and database administrator to store and manage data in a database.

Data dictionary (DD)
A repository of data elements that fully describes and locates each data element.

Data element
The raw material or individual pieces of information. These are also known as data items, fields, or attributes. These units are those that are identified in a data dictionary. These are the smallest units of data in a database.

Data file
A collection of records, often of the same type (patients, physicians, radiology, tests, etc.).

Data processing (DP)
The collection, recording, and processing of data resulting in the production of meaningful, useable information.

Data repositories and data warehouses
The electronic storage of information. In a health care organization, this includes demographic, clinical, financial, and administrative data. These repositories or warehouses may physically be in a single large, integrated database, on separate databases maintained on one computer, or on separate computers throughout the organization.

Electronic data interchange (EDI)
The electronic transmission of data used specifically to transmit business documents and correspondence over wires as opposed to through the mail.

Information
Information is data that has been processed and manipulated in a way that the results are useful and suitable for decision-making and other organizational activities.

Metadata
Data that describes the attributes of the data of a system or organization. This is the data that is stored in the data dictionary.

Record
A collection of related items of data treated as a unit. Examples include a patient in an MPI, the bill for a patient's Emergency Department visit, or a physician's pick list in the surgery system.

Structured query language (SQL)
A database query language that is used as an interface to access data on different types of database systems.

User group
All users and requesters of data.

View

A subset of the data from the database, designed for a particular user or group, giving them access to just the data and information they need.

Related Products from Opus Communications and The Greeley Company

Books

Quality Improvement Techniques for Medical Records
by Jennifer Cofer, RRA and Hugh Greeley
Provides the tips and techniques you and your staff need to successfully apply quality improvement (QI) in your department. This handbook is written specifically for medical records professionals who want to take a proactive approach to using QI tools and launch successful QI projects. You'll receive over 50 sample forms, charts, checklists, and reports that offer a solid starting point for putting your QI plan into action. In addition, you and your staff will have the opportunity to earn 8 continuing education credits simply by taking the quiz included in the book.
$47/copy, 221 pages #QMRN

Clinical Pertinence Review—Winning Strategies for Your JCAHO Survey
by Jennifer Cofer, RRA, Hugh Greeley, Monica Pappas, RRA, and Kristen Woods
Analyzes the JCAHO standards related to clinical pertinence review. This guide presents effective and efficient ways of performing each review activity—from organizing and preparing a clinical pertinence review team and selecting a representative sample of medical records to improving facility-wide medical records documentation. You'll gain essential advice on how to demonstrate compliance with JCAHO standards and present evidence of improvement to JCAHO surveyors. In addition, you and your staff will have the opportunity to earn 3 continuing education credits simply by taking the quiz included in the book.
$57/copy, 131 pages #CPRN

Information Management: The Compliance Guide to the JCAHO Standards, Second Edition
by Jennifer Cofer, RRA, Hugh Greeley, and Jay Coburn
Offers you a straightforward analysis of JCAHO's information management standards and includes detailed, practical advice on how to develop an information management plan, improve your medical records, and prepare your facility for JCAHO survey interviews. Plus, you and your staff will have the opportunity to earn 6 continuing education credits simply by taking the quiz provided in the book.
$67/copy, 140 pages #IM2N

Information Management for Home Care: The Compliance Guide to the JCAHO Standards
Designed to improve the quality of your information and presents the home care information standards in clear, easy-to-follow language. Edited by a director of quality and performance improvement and a home care information management consultant, this compliance guide helps you assess information needs and develop information strategies and policies. You'll learn how to create an information management plan, improve patient records, and prepare your agency for a JCAHO survey. In addition, this guide includes sample checklists, forms, examples, and ready-to-use advice that will make your job easier.
$67/copy, 174 pages #IMHCN

NetPractice™: A Beginner's Guide to Healthcare Networking on the Internet
by Mary Frances Miller, MS, RRA
A self-instructional guide designed to give everyone from medical staff professionals to information managers to physicians and nurses a no-nonsense approach to navigating

on the Internet. This user-friendly book doesn't try to overwhelm you with the gamut of Internet services and protocols. Instead, it lays a foundation for the most common and practical uses of the Internet—online global communications through e-mail, mailing lists, newsgroups, and the World Wide Web.
$45/copy, 234 pages #NET

Newsletters

Medical Records Briefing
Celebrating 10 years in print, *Medical Records Briefing* is a respected monthly newsletter that brings the best new ideas in health information management, plus a whole set of professional resources to benefit the medical records department. Each issue is full of crucial information, such as the latest Medicare changes, and practical advice on tough legal, financial, and human resource issues, as well as real-life success stories from other managers. Subscribers have the opportunity to earn 12 continuing education credits by successfully completing its CE quizzes, offered twice a year.
$187/year (12 issues) #MRB12

Briefings on JCAHO
The source for practical, independent guidance on succeeding in the accreditation process. Whether you're new to the survey game or are a seasoned professional, each newsletter offers quick reading and "how-to" advice on meeting JCAHO standards. For about $25 a month, readers get tips and information that otherwise could cost dearly in consulting fees and research.
$297/year (12 issues) #BOJ12

Seminars

In today's competitive marketplace, health care organizations cannot afford to waste time struggling to establish effective leadership or interpret confusing regulations from the JCAHO or other regulatory bodies. The Greeley Company offers a series of educational programs dedicated to taking the mystery out of accreditation and leadership activities. Held in hub cities across the country, these intensive, hands-on programs will provide you with easy-to-operationalize strategies and solutions to keep your organization on the cutting edge of the constantly evolving health care delivery system.

Effective JCAHO Survey Preparation
A two-day workshop for successfully complying with the JCAHO standards for hospital-based health care organizations. This successful program has helped hundreds of hospitals prepare for, achieve, and maintain Joint Commission accreditation.

Effective JCAHO Survey Preparation for Home Care Organizations
A two-day seminar designed to guide home care agencies through the challenges of preparing for a Joint Commission survey.

Effective JCAHO Survey Preparation for the Medical Staff
This unique program will provide medical staff leaders and their administrative support staff with straightforward examples of how to establish efficient monitoring and oversight of patient care quality.

Opus Communications and **The Greeley Company** are not affiliated in any way with the Joint Commission on Accreditation of Healthcare Organizations.

Order Coupon

Publication	Product #	Price	Quantity	Total
12 Weeks to a Successful Data Dictionary	DADN	$77		
QI Techniques for Medical Records	QMRN	$47		
Clinical Pertinence Review	CPRN	$57		
Information Management	IM2N	$67		
Information Management for Home Care	IMHCN	$67		
NetPractice™	NET	$45		
Medical Records Briefing	MRB12	$187/year		
Briefings on JCAHO	BOJ12	$297/year		
Shipping charges are for book purchases only. (Shipping to AK, HI, PR, and Canada is $15.)			Shipping*	$6.00
			Grand Total	

Name & Title _____
Organization _____
Street Address _____
City, State, ZIP _____
Phone _____
Fax _____
E-mail _____

❏ Check enclosed (payable to *Opus Communications*).
❏ Bill my organization. PO# _____
❏ Bill me.
❏ Bill my VISA/MasterCard/AMEX (circle one).
Account # _____ Exp. _____
Signature _____
(Your credit card bill will reflect a charge to *Opus Communications*.)

Comment Card

Please take a moment to give us your comments on *12 Weeks to a Successful Data Dictionary*. Readers' comments help us enhance our publications to meet your needs. Thank you!

_____
_____
_____
_____
_____
_____
_____
_____

You may contact me for additional information in response to my comments.
Name & Title _____
Organization _____
Street Address _____
City, State, ZIP _____
Phone _____ Fax _____
E-mail _____

Opus Communications
PO Box 1168
Marblehead, MA 01945

Phone: 800/650-6787
Fax: 800/639-8511
E-mail: customer_service@opuscomm.com
Internet: http://www.opuscomm.com

BUSINESS REPLY MAIL
FIRST CLASS MAIL   PERMIT NO 295   MARBLEHEAD MA

POSTAGE WILL BE PAID BY ADDRESSEE

OPUS COMMUNICATIONS
PO BOX 1168
MARBLEHEAD MA 01945

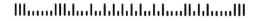

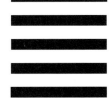

BUSINESS REPLY MAIL
FIRST CLASS MAIL   PERMIT NO 295   MARBLEHEAD MA

POSTAGE WILL BE PAID BY ADDRESSEE

OPUS COMMUNICATIONS
PO BOX 1168
MARBLEHEAD MA 01945